EXAMKRACKERS

How to Get into Medical School

A Thorough Step-by-Step Guide to Formulating Strategies for Success in the Admissions Process

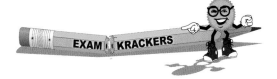

Raakhi Mohan, MD MPH

Ibrahim Busnaina, MD

ISBN 978-1-893858-50-3

1st Edition

To purchase additional copies of this book or any of the Examkrackers MCAT 5-volume set,
call 1-888-572-2536 or fax orders to 1-859-255-0109.

examkrackers.com
osote.com
audioosmosis.com

Printed and bound in China

Dedication

This is the fun part of writing a book! Of course, I'd like to dedicate my first book to my family: My mom, Aneeta, for always expecting me to put my best foot forward; My dad, Brij, for teaching me to think strategically from childhood; My sister, Mahima, for being my sounding board for everything. I appreciate your support more than you know.

—Raakhi Mohan

Many things could not have been possible without the support of my parents, Ahmed and Zainab. I'd like to dedicate my first book to them, for their unwavering support and wisdom in navigating through life.

—Ibe Busnaina

ROADMAP TO THIS BOOK

Acceptance

FREEWAY ENTRANCE

Preparation
Prerequisite Classes
Clinical Experience
Research Experience
Extracurricular
    Activities
Mental Resolve

Phase 1*
MCAT
Ordering Transcripts
AMCAS Application
Personal Statement
Letters of
    Recommendation
Researching
    Schools I**

Phase 2*
Researching
    Schools II**
Secondary
    Applications

Phase 3*
Interviews
Researching
    Schools III**
Filing Taxes
Filing FAFSA

Admissions
Decisions
Financial Aid
Researching
    Schools IV**

If you are looking for....	Go to Chapter...	Phase of Application Process
An overview of the entire application process	1: Overview of the Application Process	Any!
How to approach the prerequisites for applying to medical school (coursework, clinical experience, research, and extracurricular activities)	2: Ahead of the Game	Preparation Phase
How to approach the MCAT, AMCAS, Letters of Recommendation	3: The Primary Application	Phase 1
How to write your personal statement	4: Your Personal Statement	Phase 1
How to approach your secondaries	5: Secondary Applications	Phase 2
How to ace your interviews	6: Interviews	Phase 3
Some funny stories to make you feel good	7: Interview-day Bloopers	Phase 3
How to deal with acceptance letters and waitlists	8: Once You Start Hearing Back From Schools	Acceptance Phase

CHAPTER	CONTENTS	PAGE

1   **OVERVIEW OF THE APPLICATION PROCESS**   1

All Phases   1.1   TIMELINE & COMPONENTS OF THE APPLICATION PROCESS 1

       Figure 1.1 Components of the Application Process with Timeline   2

       1.1.1   INTRODUCTION TO PREPARATION PHASE 4

          Figure 1.1.1 Setting Goals for the Admissions Process 5

       1.1.2   PHASE 1 INTRODUCTION 5

          Figure 1.1.2 MCAT Format & Scoring 7

       1.1.3   PHASE 2 INTRODUCTION 7

       1.1.4   PHASE 3 INTRODUCTION 8

       1.1.5   INTRODUCTION TO ACCEPTANCE PHASE 9

   1.2   KEY PLAYERS IN THE ADMISSIONS PROCESS.............................. 9

       1.2.1   UNDERGRADUATE PREMED COMMITTEE 9

       1.2.2   MEDICAL SCHOOL ADMISSIONS COMMITTEES 10

       1.2.3   EVERY INTERACTION COUNTS 10

   1.3   NON-TRADITIONAL APPLICANTS 11

2   **AHEAD OF THE GAME**   13

Preparation Phase   2.1   WHEN TO START PLANNING 13

   2.2   WHAT ARE MEDICAL SCHOOLS LOOKING FOR? PREPARING TO APPLY 14

       2.2.1   COURSEWORK & MAJORS 14

       2.2.2   PREMED PREREQUISITES 15

       2.2.3   EXTRACURRICULAR ACTIVITIES 16

       2.2.4   RESEARCH 17

       2.2.5   CLINICAL EXPERIENCE 19

   2.3   NON-TRADITIONAL APPLICANTS 22

3   **PRIMARY APPLICATION**   23

Phase 1   3.1   SIGNIFICANCE 23

   3.2   IDENTIFYING INFORMATION 24

       3.2.1   DISADVANTAGED STATUS 24

          Figure 3.2.1 Sample Disadvantaged Mini-Statement 25-6

       3.22   INSTITUTIONAL ACTION 27

   3.3   DESIGNATING COURSES FOR YOUR SCIENCE GPA (BCPM DESIGNATION) 27

   3.4   WORK & ACTIVITIES 29

   3.5   LETTERS OF RECOMMENDATION 31

       3.5.1   WHO TO ASK 31

       3.5.2   MAKING THE REQUEST 32

   3.6   RESEARCHING SCHOOLS I (SELECTING RECIPIENT SCHOOLS) 33

   3.7   MD-PHD APPLICANTS 34

4	**YOUR PERSONAL STATEMENT**		**37**
Phase 1	4.1	BEFORE YOU BEGIN...	37
		4.1.1 PURPOSE OF THE PERSONAL STATEMENT	37
	4.2	THE 'FIVE GOLDEN STEPS' TO CONQUERING YOUR PERSONAL STATEMENT	38
		4.2.1 STEP 1: THE FIRST 2 'CARDINAL QUESTIONS'	38
		Figure 4.2.1 Sample Cardinal Question Brainstorm	39
		4.2.2 STEP 2: CONSTRUCTING A 'SELF-REFLECTION CHART'	39
		Figure 4.2.2a: What is a Self-Reflection Chart?	42
		Figure 4.2.2b: Sample Completed Self-Reflection Chart	44
		4.2.3 STEP 3: CONNECTING THE DOTS	45
		Figure 4.2.3a: Sample Connect-the-Dots	46
		Figure 4.2.3b: Sample Self-Reflection Chart with Selected Topics & Connect-the-Dots	47
		4.2.4 STEP 4: CHOOSE YOUR 'GIFT WRAP'	48
		4.2.5 STEP 5: OUTLINE!	50
		Figure 4.2.5a: Sample Outline	51
		Figure 4.2.5b: Sample Personal Statement	52-3
	4.3	THE WRITING PROCESS—ANTICIPATING ROADBLOCKS	53
		4.3.1 PARAGRAPH STRUCTURE	53
		4.3.2 LENGTH	54
		4.3.3 QUOTES	55
		4.3.4 IMAGERY	56
		4.3.5 THE FUDGE FACTOR	57
		4.3.6 GRAMMAR REFRESHER	58
		4.3.7 TONE & FLOW	61
		4.3.8 PROOFREADING	62
	4.4	GIVING YOURSELF ENOUGH TIME	63
	4.5	NON-TRADITIONAL APPLICANTS	64
		Figure 4.5 Sample Non-traditional Essay	65-7
5	**THE SECONDARY APPLICATION**		**69**
Phase 2	5.1	HOW IMPORTANT ARE THEY?	69
		5.1.1 EXAMPLES OF SOME COMMON SECONDARY QUESTIONS	69
	5.2	HOW TO TACKLE SECONDARIES	69
		5.2.1 REFERRING BACK	70
		5.2.2 RESEARCHING SCHOOLS II (INSTITUTION-TARGETED RESPONSES)	70
		5.2.3 SHORT & SWEET	71
		5.2.4 LET YOUR PERSONALITY SHINE THROUGH	72
	5.3	MAXIMIZING EFFICACY OF SECONDARIES	72

Phase 3

6.1   NAILING YOUR INTERVIEW **73**
     6.1.1   THE IMPORTANCE OF INTERVIEW PERFORMANCE 73
     6.1.2   WHAT IS A 'SALES PITCH'? 74

6.2   THE 'SIX PLATINUM STEPS' TO A SAVVY SALES PITCH **74**
     6.2.1   STEP 1: REVIEW YOUR BRAINSTORM FOR THE CARDINAL QUESTIONS 74
         Figure 6.2.1a: Cheyenne's Brainstorm to the
         First 2 Cardinal Questions 75
     6.2.2   STEP 2: THE THIRD CARDINAL QUESTION:
         WHAT DO YOU WANT TO ACCOMPLISH IN MEDICINE? 75
         Figure 6.2.2 Sample Brainstorm to the Third Cardinal Question 76
     6.2.3   STEP 3: PUT ANSWERS TO THE THREE CARDINAL QUESTIONS
         IN STORY FORM 76
         Figure 6.2.3a Sample Story Developed from Answers to the
         Three Cardinal Questions 77-9
         Figure 6.2.3b Alternate Storyline 79-80
     6.2.4   STEP 4: ADD 'FLAVA'! 80
         Figure 6.2.4 Sample of Weaving Additional Self-Reflection Chart
         Contents into Story 81
     6.2.5   STEP 5: BE ABLE TO TELL THE WHOLE STORY IN 5 MINUTES OR 50 81
     6.2.6   CUSTOMIZE YOUR PITCH FOR EACH SCHOOL (RESEARCHING SCHOOLS III) .. 82
         Figure 6.2.6a Sample Sales-Pitch Customization 84
         Figure 6.2.6b Cheyenne's Self-Reflection Chart 85-6
         Figure 6.2.6c Table of Online Resources 86

6.3   DELIVERING THE PITCH **87**

6.4   SHOULD I BE DOING ANYTHING ELSE TO PREPARE? **93**

6.5   TIPS FOR SUCCESS **94**
     6.5.1   GETTING INTO THE RIGHT MINDSET 94
     6.5.2   GROUP INTERVIEWS 95
     6.5.3   MULTIPLE INTERVIEWS 95
     6.5.4   DON'T LET YOUR GUARD DOWN! 96
     6.5.5   FOLLOW UP 96
     6.5.6   APPEARANCE, MAINTENANCE, AND LOGISTICS 96
         Figure 6.5.6 Appearance, Maintenance, and Logistics 96-7

6.6   WHAT IS INTERVIEW DAY LIKE? **97**
     6.6.1   THE STRUCTURE OF THE DAY 97
     6.6.2   TAKE NOTES! 101
     6.6.3   EXPECT TOUGH QUESTIONS 101

6.7   NON-TRADITIONAL APPLICANTS **105**

7	**INTERVIEW DAY BLOOPERS**	107

Phase 3

7.1	MURPHY'S LAW	107
7.2	STORY 1	108
7.3	STORY 2	109
7.4	STORY 3	110
7.5	STORY 4	111

8	**ONCE YOU START HEARING BACK FROM SCHOOLS**	113

Acceptance Phase

8.1	HOW LONG SHOULD I WAIT BEFORE SAYING 'YES!'	113
8.2	DO I HAVE ANY HOPE ON A WAITLIST?	114
8.3	LEVERAGING OFFERS	116
8.4	DEFERRING ADMISSIONS	117
8.5	FINANCIAL AID PACKAGES	118
8.6	RESEARCHING SCHOOLS IV	119
8.5.1	CURRICULUM	119
8.5.2	THE BOARDS	120
8.5.3	RESIDENCY MATCH	120
8.5.4	STRENGTHS IN YOUR AREAS OF INTEREST	121
8.5.5	LIFESTYLE	121

A	**APPENDIX**	123

A.1	OUR MED-SCHOOL SLANG: GLOSSARY OF TERMINOLOGY	123
A.2	APPLICATION TIMELINE: OVERVIEW	125-6

G	**GLOSSARY**	127

ALLOPATHIC SCHOOLS	127
NATROPATHIC SCHOOLS	200
OSTEOPATHIC SCHOOLSS	203

ABOUT THE AUTHORS	215

USEFUL ONLINE RESOURCES*

MCAT

http://www.aamc.org/students/mcat/start.htm

http://www.examkrackers.com

http://www.aamc.org/students/applying/start.htm

Researching Schools I

http://www.aamc.org/data/facts

http://www.usnews.com

http://en.wikipedia.org/wiki/University_ranking

http://grants2.nih.gov/grants/award/trends/medschc.htm

http://services.aamc.org/currdir/section2/start.cfm (joint degree)

Personal Statement

http://www.aamc.org/students/amcas/start.htm

Researching Schools II

Individual Schools' Websites

Partial Index:
http://www.usnews.com/usnews/edu/grad/directory/dir-med/dirmedindex_brief.php

Researching Schools III

http://services.aamc.org/currdir/section2/start.cfm (curricula)

Acceptance Phase

http://services.aamc.org/tsfreports/

*Listing of online resources in the above and subsequent resource tables is provided for information purposes only and implies no endorsement on the part of the authors. These web links are live and operating as of this publication, and are subject to change.

PREFACE

Book's Intention

Much of the logistical information for applicants in the text of this book refers to U.S. allopathic medical schools using the AMCAS application system. However, we recognize that there are many schools that don't fit into this category: allopathic schools not using AMCAS, osteopathic schools, naturopathic schools, and foreign medical schools. Our tips on the personal statement and interview are applicable to all applicants, and our advice on the primary application is easily translated to a first-round application to a non-AMCAS or non-allopathic medical school. Here is a brief list of services used by other U.S. medical schools not mentioned in the text of this book; much of what we have written will still apply, and AMCAS-related tips can normally be replaced with any of the systems listed below.

TMDSAS

TEXAS MEDICAL AND DENTAL SCHOOL APPLICATION SERVICE
www.utsystem.edu/tmdsas

This service is used chiefly by the University of Texas medical schools, except in some circumstances for MD/PhD applicants. MCAT scores and transcripts need to be submitted separately to this system and additional fees must bepaid.

AACOMAS

AMERICAN ASSOCIATION OF COLLEGES OF OSTEOPATHIC MEDICINE APPLICATION SERVICE
https://aacomas.aacom.org

This service is used for applications to osteopathic schools in the United States, with the exception of the Texas College of Osteopathic medicine (which uses TMDSAS). Again, MCAT scores and transcripts must be sent manually to this service, and primary and secondary application fees apply. In general, when applying to osteopathic schools it is strongly recommended that you emphasize why osteopathic medicine (as opposed to allopathic) is your choice (don't say it's a back-up!), and some schools require at least one letter of recommendation from a DO (Doctor of Osteopathy).

Early Decision

Most medical schools offer the option of applying for early decision. However, unlike the case with undergraduate schools, early decision does not tend to confer a statistical advantage upon applicants. It remains very difficult to be admitted to a medical school via early decision, and applicants are unable to apply simultaneously in the regular application cycle until a decision is rendered on the early application, which does not happen before October 1st. This puts applicants who aren't admitted early in a bind and at a distinct disadvantage if they have to scramble to put together a regular AMCAS application by October 15th. Unless you have a compelling reason for setting your sights on one particular institution, and have a strong, solid academic record, early decision may not be your best option.

Combined Programs

So, you're way ahead of the game! A few institutions offer combined BA-MD programs that admit a select number of students from the undergraduate side of the university directly into the medical school. Typically, these programs attach GPA and MCAT conditions to their acceptances, making final admission contingent on maintaining minimums in both categories (typically higher than what they would accept from regular AMCAS season applicants). These programs usually allow participants to major in whatever they wish, as long as they fulfill the premedical requirements. To get into one of these programs, you must apply either out of high school or during your freshman or sophomore year. Most of these programs require an interview, even if you are a current student. Also, if you apply to such a program as a freshman or sophomore, you have to have been following the premed track from the start in order to be on schedule. Each school has different requirements and processes, so you should do some research. Schools offering this track include Northwestern, USC, NYU, Brown, and Boston University. Keep in mind, however, that although these programs may fast-track you into med school, many also condense undergrad and med school so that you lose a year to enjoy just being a college student.

International Students (Non-U.S. Citizens or Permanent Residents)

Even if you have attended a U.S. undergraduate institution and are an exceptional applicant, if you are not a U.S. citizen or permanent resident it is difficult to gain admission to a U.S. medical school. Unfortunately, as U.S. medical schools are extremely expensive and financial aid comes primarily from federal funding, which can only be received by U.S. citizens and permanent residents, medical schools are hesitant to consider international applicants. Some schools will not even consider applications submitted by international students, many schools will. The ones that do may require admitted international students to establish an escrow account containing enough funds to cover four years of tuition in order to matriculate. If medical school in the United States is beyond your financial reach, you may consider just doing residency in America to get a U.S. license. Many medical schools abroad are state-funded and allow you to pursue residency in the United States by taking additional exams; this may be a more realistic option.

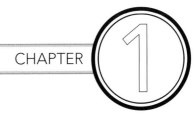

Overview of the Application Process

1.1 Timeline & Components of the Application Process

The medical school application process is rather involved and time-consuming. Heck, if it weren't so complex, we wouldn't need to write a book to help you successfully navigate the process. We've divided up the various stages of this process into a **preparation** period, three phases of the **actual application process**, and then a period for making **acceptance decisions**. This organization is based on the timeline of the application process, and includes facets that most people don't talk about.

For example, getting official transcripts from all of your post-secondary schools is a time-consuming task, and often an expensive one. Even though this step is often overlooked, you will need to allot time and money to it—so we discuss it in this book. Our list is comprehensive; all applicants to U.S. allopathic medical schools will have to engage in each of these components of the application process.

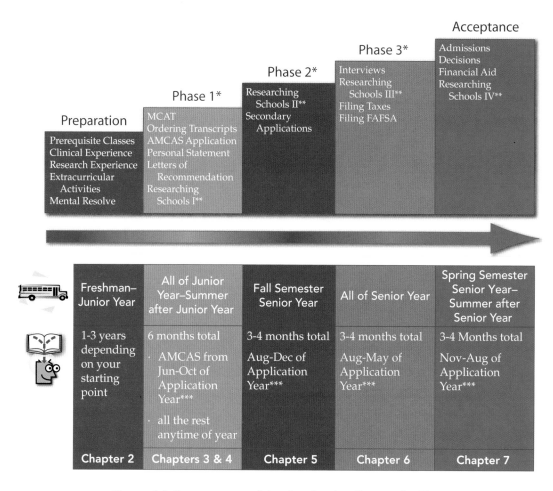

Figure 1.1 Components of the Application Process by Phase
with Timeline for Traditional and Nontraditional Applicants

*You determine your own pace through this process! These phases of the process last as long as it takes for you to complete the tasks within them. If you are really efficient, and start early, you could move from Phase 1 to Acceptance in just five months. Different people require different amounts of time to complete all these components-plan at a pace that is realistic for you. In order to arrange a realistic schedule, you'll have to honestly consider factors such as your work style, which application components will be the most challenging for you, and other responsibilities requiring your time and energy during this process.

**Researching Schools I-IV: you may be wondering what this is all about and why you can't just research schools once. Well, the fact is that you will want to know about different aspects of schools at different phases of the application process. When deciding whether to apply to a particular school, you will want to research the profile of their average accepted student to know what your chances of admission would be. You may also wish to consider the school's ranking and location at this phase (Phase 1). However, when you are tailoring your secondary applications (Phase 2), you will need to focus your research on what strengths the school has and how those align with your goals in medicine. Finally, when deciding to accept an offer for an interview (Phase 3) or admission (Phase 4), you will want to research aspects of the school that increase the probability of your being happy and successful there, such as their residency-match rate, board-passing rates, and average graduate debt. Jumping around is not advisable; for example, it's a waste of your time and energy (which the application process already demands a lot of!) to engage in Phase 3 school research when you are canvassing schools in Phase I. Some helpful resources for the different phases of research are listed in a quick reference table at the beginning of this book, and we go into further detail in the relevant chapters.

***The "Application Year"** is tailored to the school year, and thus spans approximately from one summer to the next. The earliest you can begin applying is June of any given year, and the process cannot extend past the following August, 14 months later. Most applicants do not take a whole year as the application process involves rolling admissions, in which those who apply first will hear back first. So if you start in June by submitting your Phase 1 materials, you will likely hear back from schools early and know your outcome by early spring. If you start later in the fall, your process may extend into the following summer.

Throughout this book, we've used icons to help you quickly identify and refer back to various sections. Below is an explanation of what these icons represent:

Non-traditional Applicants: In general, everything in this book applies to you. We provide you with strategies for getting accepted rather than just logistical information. In the non-traditional applicant sections at the end of each chapter, we address additional considerations.

Traditional Applicants: Anyone who has taken the premed prerequisites, and who is applying to medical school in his or her junior year of college, is considered a traditional applicant.

Recycle: Putting the pieces of the process together in order to maximize your time and energy by utilizing the same tools throughout the application process.

Road Hazard! Flags tips for avoiding common mistakes and pitfalls in the application process.

The Zen Factor: Flags tips on how to approach the different components of the process with the right mindset.

1.1.1 Introduction to Preparation Phase

You may be wondering why we have a section on preparing to apply. Well, the average medical school aspirant has two to three years of work to do in order to apply. You really have to be mentally prepared to follow through with your decision. Not that everyone who applies to medical school (or who actually goes to medical school) is 110% sure of his or her decision, but you should be above 80%, just to ensure that going through this process is worth it. If you are not sure, a good way to start is to get some exposure to clinical medicine and to see if you can deal with the tough basic science classes. In addition to possessing this mental resolve, you will need to take about eight semesters' worth of prerequisite classes and be able to demonstrate valuable exposure to clinical medicine and research, just to be able to apply. Strategies for these components of the preparation phase are delineated in Chapter 2: Ahead of the Game.

These days medical schools can be choosier about whom they accept—there are plenty of qualified candidates. Being a doctor in the twenty-first century involves a great deal of interpersonal communication skills. In addition to treating your patients, you will need to be able to educate, empathize, and even negotiate with them. From your own experiences of being sick, you can understand that patients are often scared and uncomfortable, and therefore not always pleasant to deal with. Furthermore, medicine often involves serious ethical dilemmas. Unless you go into radiology, communication and demeanor are going to play an important role in your daily life. Medical schools want to make sure you can handle this aspect of the job. Applicants with more personality (whether it's a great sense of humor or a hard-core passion for a certain research topic) are considered more personable and patient-friendly. For this reason, medical schools have been accepting more and more non-traditional students over the last decade. Non-science undergraduate degrees, previous non-medical careers, achievements in the arts, and foreign-travel experience are characteristics more commonly found in matriculating med students. It's not that you must possess these elements to get in, but the strengthening correlation of these attributes to acceptance shows how the bar is being raised: now, not only do you have to make the grade, but you also have to be well-rounded (or at least easy to talk to).

The Spectrum of Premedness

Different people have different expectations concerning this process. Some will be relieved just to get an acceptance, while others will shun offers from any school that is not a top-ten. Below is a rough guide for three tracks to get into medical school. It is best used as a tool to set your targets for the journey ahead of you. A top-ten school may accept an applicant who has an MCAT score below 30—an application is, after all, a gestalt. And conversely, we've seen 4.0 students with MCAT scores in the 40s denied admission. However, this is rare. The numbers below are thresholds to delineate high-probability territory.

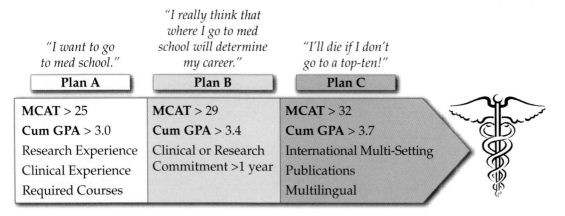

"I want to go to med school."	"I really think that where I go to med school will determine my career."	"I'll die if I don't go to a top-ten!"
Plan A	**Plan B**	**Plan C**
MCAT > 25	MCAT > 29	MCAT > 32
Cum GPA > 3.0	**Cum GPA** > 3.4	**Cum GPA** > 3.7
Research Experience	Clinical or Research Commitment >1 year	International Multi-Setting
Clinical Experience		Publications
Required Courses		Multilingual

Figure 1.1.1 Setting Goals for the Admission Process

1.1.2   Phase 1 Introduction

AMCAS

AMCAS is the infamous American Medical College Application Service, which is run by the AAMC (Association of American Medical Colleges). The application is completely online, although you have to arrange for each of your post-secondary schools to send AMCAS transcripts directly. The process of sending your transcripts, work history, extracurricular activities, and personal statement to medical schools through AMCAS is called your Primary Application (Chapter 3).

The most time-consuming aspect of the primary application is the personal statement (Chapter 4); it doesn't take much time to write one page, but when you have only one page in which to provide medical schools with a window into your soul, the task becomes trickier. The personal statement, called "personal comments" by AMCAS, is a crucial part of your primary. While the majority of schools will concentrate on your GPA and MCAT score in their first run through applications, the decision to offer an applicant a secondary application or interview is often heavily based on the personal statement (especially for applicants who have GPAs and MCAT scores that fall among or below the mean values for applicants).

MCAT

MCAT is the Medical College Admissions Test, which is also run by the AAMC. The primary application may be submitted before you take the MCAT; however, many schools will not even look at your application until they receive your MCAT scores. The MCAT is now administered about 22 times a year, and can be retaken three times any given year. The schools will see all of your MCAT scores in your Testing History Report, so you really should not take the exam until you are scoring within your target range on your practice tests.

The test was intended to provide a more standardized reflection of an applicant's scholastic aptitude than GPA, as grading systems vary widely among colleges. However, as in most standardized tests, an applicant's performance depends just as much on his or her test-taking strategy as it does on his or her scholastic aptitude. For this reason, it really is a good idea to take an MCAT prep course. Another good reason to study from MCAT prep course books is that they condense the material you need to focus on and offer several helpful short-cuts to memorization and strategy. Further details of the exam are outlined in the table below. The MCAT consists of four sections:

1. **Physical Sciences** (undergraduate physics and inorganic chemistry)

2. **Verbal Reasoning** (a variety of passage topics, most intentionally soporific, ranging from economics and anthropology to poetic analysis)

3. **Writing Sample** (two essays on given topics)

4. **Biological Sciences** (a wide range of undergraduate biology topics, organic chemistry, and genetics)

Test Section	Questions	Time Allotted	Time/Question
Tutorial	(Optional)	10 minutes	
Physical Sciences	52	70 minutes	~1.35 minutes (81s)
Break	(Optional)	10 minutes	
Verbal Reasoning	40	60 minutes	1.5 minutes (90s)
Break	(Optional)	10 minutes	
Writing Sample	2	60 minutes	30 minutes/essay
Break	(Optional)	10 minutes	
Biological Sciences	52	70 minutes	~1.35 minutes (81s)
Survey		10 minutes	
Total Content Time		4 hours, 20 minutes	
Total Test Time		**5 hours, 10 minutes**	

Figure 1.1.2 MCAT Format & Scoring

Researching Schools I

This is your first round of research on medical schools. At this point in the process, most applicants are pretty nervous about getting in. Your purpose in researching schools right now is to answer the question, "Should I apply here?" There are hundreds medical schools around the country, and you don't want to apply to all of them. We'll provide some simple, realistic strategies that will help you choose from among them.

1.1.3   Phase 2 Introduction

'Secondaries'

Secondary applications (Chapter 6) are another way for schools to pare down their applicant pool. In some cases, receiving a supplementary application is a good sign, and you should be excited because you are more likely to be offered an interview. Most secondaries are essay-response questions, with more and more schools trending toward multiple short-answer essay questions. These essays usually allow you to elaborate on topics you had to condense in your primary application, such as a clinical experience or academic achievement. Secondaries are also an opportunity for schools to make money, so it's no surprise that secondary application fees are common.

Let's face it, everyone has heard a horror story of someone with a great GPA and MCAT score who still didn't get in. Just try to remember that there are plenty of applicants with non-Herculean scores that do get accepted.

Researching Schools II

A key strategy to handling these supplemental applications is to tailor them to the individual schools, which you cannot do in Phase I. The school has taken a step forward in selecting you to progress to Phase 2, so you need to reciprocate by letting them know you are also interested in them. Your secondary essays are not going to be eulogies on how much you love the school, but they should demonstrate an interest in some aspect of the school. Thus, this round of research involves looking at what facets of the school you like. AAMC provides a wealth of resources on schools, with tables on school curricula types, minority enrollment, etc. School websites are great for finding out program strengths, latest news, and achievements, etc. This round of research is short and sweet—you just need to find something to incorporate into your application that shows the school that you are tuned into their particular institution.

1.1.4   Phase 3 Introduction

Interviews

The admissions interview is the most feared component of the application process by far. This is understandable because preparing for an interview is a nebulous task, unlike the MCAT, for which you can memorize information and take practice tests. Furthermore, premed students usually don't have much experience in job-interviewing and marketing themselves. In Chapter 7, we walk you through the basics of how to market yourself (and to be comfortable about it) during the admissions interview. You have to walk in to the interview with a clear idea of what facets of your background, personality, and motivations make you a great candidate.

Researching Schools III

The interview is also an important opportunity for you to see if this is truly a school you would like to attend. Almost all interviewers will allow time for you to ask them questions about the institution. The more informed your questions, the more it shows your interest in the school. At the same time, you want to ask questions about things that really matter to you. So, in this round of research, you really want to think about what factors would make you happy and successful at a given institution. It's okay not to have questions! A lot of applicants think it's a faux pas not to have a super insightful question. The point is to show your interviewer that you are genuinely interested in attending the institution and aren't just interviewing there because it's fun or because you want the practice. In Chapter 6, we'll show you how to weave this round of research into your interview strategy.

Another important, yet often overlooked, reason for this round of research is to decide whether you want to accept an interview. Many candidates receive several interview invitations and need to be selective because travelling for an interview can be very expensive! Since this round of research focuses on your potential happiness and success at a given school, this is also a good time to revisit how you have prioritized schools. This will help you to make your decision should you be offered multiple acceptances.

1.1.5   Introduction to Acceptance Phase
You may be wondering why there is a phase allotted for acceptance. Most applicants are focused on just getting in somewhere and see an acceptance letter as the endpoint. In reality, the whole process involves you prioritizing your options, just as the med schools prioritize in their ranking of applicants. In Chapter 8, we'll walk you through the three important issues in this phase: how to handle being waitlisted, what to look for in your financial aid offer, and choosing a school.

1.2 KEY PLAYERS IN THE ADMISSIONS PROCESS

1.2.1   Undergraduate Premed Committee
Most colleges have an undergraduate pre-health, or premed, committee which helps to coordinate their students' medical school recommendation letters. Often, teachers will send their recommendation letters to the premed committee, who will then form a composite letter that is more comprehensive. These committees were first formed in part because science teachers didn't always have the greatest skills in writing impressive recommendation letters (big surprise), and applications were suffering. With premed committees, the scientists can write what they like about you, and the committees can select the best parts from all of your recommendation letters. They combine these highlights with information they gather on you to form a composite that is a much stronger recommendation.

Different premed committees offer different services; some help you to edit your personal statement, others even offer practice interview sessions. You should check with your school to see whether it has a premed committee and what services it provides. In particular, it is helpful to know whether your premed committee ranks applicants in their communications to medical schools. We have heard of applicants who opt to circumvent the premed committee out of fear of having their rank conveyed to medical schools. If you opt not to have a committee composite letter written, medical schools tend to interpret this as an indication of your having skeletons to hide. If your academic record is solid and you don't have any major disciplinary issues, it simply isn't worth the risk to bypass the committee.

1.2.2 Medical School Admissions Committees

U.S. allopathic medical schools process approximately 40,000-50,000 applications every year. You can imagine what a gargantuan task this is. Instead of hiring a ton of admissions staff, schools form admissions committees for free. Many professors, residents, and current medical (usually 4th-year) students volunteer their time to be on these committees because they care about the quality of the incoming class; others must sit on these committees to fulfill contractual obligations. Of course, admissions staff are also included.

Most admissions committees will divide up into teams or pairs, which then receive a portion of the applications to review. In this manner, they divvy up the workload while ensuring that each application is reviewed by more than one person. The teams will then report back to the whole committee, with a recommendation of how to proceed on each application they reviewed. Other committee members have a chance to ask questions, bring up concerns, or present their opinions, and then the whole committee makes a consensus decision. For each phase of the admissions process, an application can be filed as a "go," a "no," or a "maybe."

1.2.3 Every Interaction Counts

Remember how we said that admissions committees include admissions staff? This means you really have to be on your best behavior any time you interact with the Admissions Office. If you irritate the secretary, there is a chance that she will bring this up in a committee meeting. Similarly, medical students that give tours of schools say they are not affiliated with the admissions departments—they are just volunteers. However, they interface with the department before and after every tour, so you can imagine that if someone made a bad impression, gossip may easily spread. For example, an applicant once expressed great surprise at metal detectors in a county hospital during an interview tour, and then commented on how he had never worked in a public-care setting. The tour guide happened to mention the incident to a physician on the admissions committee during casual conversation, joking that the applicant would probably have a tough time adjusting to a county general hospital. The physician brought this up when the applicant's file was being reviewed by the committee, and the applicant was viewed as less likely to fit in to the school. This may sound a bit Zen, but you really should put forward only positive energy surrounding your application. Similarly, how well you treat the secretary of the premed committee could result in your letters being sent out to the AAMC on time.

1.3 NON-TRADITIONAL APPLICANTS

Not that this is any surprise to you, but you have a little more work to do than the straight-out-of-undergrad applicant. Statistics have shown that 20-30% of applicants over 24 are admitted to medical school, while 45% of 21 to 23-year-olds are. However, given that you've probably pursued other interests, you may be clearer in your decision to apply to med school than other applicants. The good news is that medical schools welcome the maturity non-traditional applicants tend to exude in their applications and interviews, as well as the experience and perspective gained from simply having a more varied life story.

About half of the applicants to U.S. allopathic schools today have taken time off, pursued another graduate degree, or followed another career path before making the decision to enter medicine. So, as a non-traditional applicant, you don't have to worry about being an exception or needing special consideration; non-traditional applicants aren't really in the minority anymore.

One of the benefits of this is that the application process is exactly the same for non-traditional and traditional applicants. The extra work for non-traditional applicants arises from the logistics involved. For example, you may have a more difficult time getting your science grades accepted, getting academic letters of recommendation, and studying for the MCAT if you graduated college a few years ago. Many schools will allow alumni to access their premed committees during the application process, so non-traditional students should contact their undergraduate institutions to inquire. In addition to the services discussed above, premed committees will help you to work progressively through the process with their deadlines and communications. Plus, they can answer questions and help you to feel less alone through the application process, as you may not know anyone else who is applying at the same time.

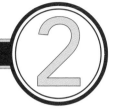

AHEAD OF THE GAME

2.1 WHEN TO START PLANNING

Congratulations! You've made the decision to pursue a career in medicine. One of the most difficult parts of the process is over. Some applicants enter undergrad knowing they want to go to medical school; others make the decision years after graduating. Since the majority of applicants apply while in their junior year of college, those applying to medical school after this time are considered 'non-traditional applicants,' whom we discuss at the end of this chapter.

Applications are usually submitted during the fall of the senior year, so applicants usually begin the application process during the summer between junior and senior year. Since most application deadlines are right at the beginning of the senior year, you really only have freshman through junior year to squeeze in pre-requisites and activities to impress admissions committees. If you are reading this in your second semester junior year, or are a senior who's going to take a year off, you're right on schedule with beginning the application process. If you are in your senior year, and you are not taking a year off, you may want to just skip to the most relevant chapter for you (e.g. Go right to the personal statement chapter (**Chapter 4**) if you need to get your statement done ASAP).

39,108 applicants in 2006—only 17,370 matriculated. That's only 44.4%! Use the tips in this chapter to get ahead of the game.

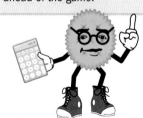

For a general timeline of the admissions process, refer back to **Appendix A. 2**. Don't worry if you're a bit ahead or behind. If you're just thinking about being pre-med, skimming this book now will give you a good idea of what lies ahead, so you can begin (at least subconsciously) making strategic decisions. At the same time, worrying seriously about any of this before junior year is definitely not worth it; you'll have plenty to keep you busy and you'll be surprised how much you change from freshman to junior year.

2.2 What are Medical Schools Looking For? Preparing to Apply

2.2.1 Coursework & Majors

Planning your undergraduate course load can be confusing and overwhelming. Depending on when you made your decision to apply to med school, you may have total or somewhat limited flexibility. Regardless of when you made the decision, though, you should remember one thing: do what makes you happy. Don't take courses just because you think you should or because you think doing so will impress medical school admissions committees. What will impress admissions committees is a *demonstrated commitment to something* about which you care deeply; this could be anything from acting in a television sitcom to volunteering in a hospice. The same rule goes for coursework. Beyond what is absolutely required for medical school, your major and elective choice are up to you. The only exception is if you did poorly in a pre-med requirement course (B or below); in this case, you should take, and perform well in, an upper-level science course to demonstrate that you can handle the rigor of medical school's standard basic science curriculum.

You can major in anything your heart desires, as long as you complete the medical school prerequisite classes. The question that haunts many pre-meds is, Should I major in a science? Well, pragmatically speaking, majoring in a science will make the first year or two of medical school a bit easier. If you major in biology, biochemistry, chemistry, or a more specialized discipline incorporating any of these three, you should not have much trouble with many of the required basic science exams. However, you'll miss out on all that other knowledge that you can't acquire in medical school—college is one of the few times in your life where you can, and should, study whatever interests you. Another consideration is the opportunity to study abroad; majoring in a science at many universities makes it difficult for students to study abroad.

Medical schools accept plenty of people who majored in non-sciences; in fact, they accept roughly the same percentage of science and non-science majors. Recall that the requirements for every applicant include completing the pre-med requirements, as well as demonstrating that you can handle the rigors of medical school. The latter can be demonstrated by doing well in the required classes and upper-level science courses, or doing well on the science sections of the MCAT.

2.2.2 Pre-med Prerequisites

Note: These courses may differ slightly between schools.

Math	Calculus, 2 semesters
	Statistics, 1 semester
Biology	Introductory Biology with Lab, 2 semesters
Chemistry	General (Inorganic) Chemistry with Lab, 2 semesters
	Organic Chemistry with Lab, 2 semesters
Physics	(can be calculus or non-calculus based), 2 semesters
English	2 semesters

The truth is that many of the prerequisites are not really subjects you have to excel in to be a good doctor. If you asked most doctors to perform an integral, or delineate an Sn^2 reaction, they would be about as blank as you may feel right now. The prerequisites are intended to weed out those who do not have the tenacity to master a difficult subject. Almost half of all students who enter college as premeds change their minds because of their suffering in a premed prerequisite class. In this manner, the medical institution maintains high barriers to entry, and thus a 'quality control' of sorts. Ideal medical candidates demonstrate a well-cultivated desire to be doctors by jumping gracefully through the hoops of the medical admissions process. So, in general, you need to do well in these classes.

Unfortunately, it's really hard to excel in the hardest subjects, especially since you will likely be taking more than one at a time. Here's a tip: take a few of these courses at a community college where they may be less challenging. Medical schools don't care if you take a summer of physics at a community college to complete the two semester requirement, or take it at Harvey Mudd College (where it's super challenging). You won't be able to take all of your prerequisites at a community college—there are too many to take, and medical schools have wised up to this practice. However, you can figure out which prerequisite couses terrify you most and try to take them in a less threatening environment. It's always better if the credits are transferable to your primary school, which usually isn't a problem.

Keep in mind that the more comfortable you are in these subjects, the easier your preparation for the MCAT will be, as well as your coursework in the first years of medical school. However, the truth is you won't use that much calculus after you take that prerequisite, and the same is true of many of the others. Another strategy is to take an MCAT prep course, and even the MCAT, before a difficult prerequisite. This way, you can get an introduction to the main concepts in organic chemistry, for example, before you take it for a grade at school. This is not a bad idea for physics, organic chemistry, anatomy, physiology, and many other science classes.

2.2.3 Extracurricular Activities

Okay, so you have all this stuff to do just to be able to *apply* to medical school. However, just because medicine may be your career, it doesn't have to be your entire life. So take some time to enjoy yourself. Non-medical extracurricular activities are important, not only to maintain your sanity, but to demonstrate that you have social skills. Medical schools are trending toward accepting more well-rounded applicants, so diversify your portfolio, so to speak. The reason behind this is important. Medical schools used to incentivize excellence in the hard sciences, so they were churning out doctors that were mostly science dorks with few people skills. Now, medical institutions have learned that people who spend most of their time with test tubes may not be the best at communicating with their patients. A person who aces organic chemistry will not necessarily be emotionally sensitive during challenging patient interactions.

So how can a medical school determine if you have decent interpersonal skills? On paper, it's through your extracurricular activities. Non-medical extracurricular activities represent a great opportunity for demonstrating leadership skills that medical schools value. The medical field views doctors as leaders in society and seeks to uphold that reputation. So they look fondly upon people who have started their own projects or clubs, or who hold leadership positions in established clubs. Sticking with an activity, and achieving greater responsibility over time, looks great. Schools appreciate long-term commitment because, well, becoming a doctor requires a long-term commitment. For this reason, those of you who love to play sports should keep doing so (even if it's just on an intramural team).

In addition to leadership, applicants active in the humanities are thought to have greater patient skills. In other words, the medical institution has learned that applicants who are cultured, well-traveled, or involved in the arts tend to have more solid interpersonal communication skills. It may seem as though the medical institution's emphasis on patient interaction is a bit overblown. But it isn't. Research is clear that the when doctor-patient interaction is good the level of health care is better, patients are more compliant with treatment and prevention services, and fewer malpractice suits are filed. Anyone that has been sick understands that patients feel vulnerable, and oftentimes scared. From the patient's perspective, it is almost as important to be able to acknowledge and attend to the patient's feelings and fears as it is to give him or her medical attention. Many medical schools have gone through the trouble of adding to their curricula a class that focuses on doctor-patient interaction. However, it's easier for a school to turn out top-notch doctors if it has students who are already well versed in interpersonal communications.

You can, and should, choose activities which will help you to work on weaknesses in your application. For example, if you know you are really shy and scared of public speaking, try taking an acting or communications class. Similarly, you can view extracurricular activities as a way to highlight certain skills strategically. For example, if you want to emphasize your leadership abilities, running for student government may be a good idea. But don't engage in an activity just because you think it will look good to an admissions committee! You already have all those classes, the MCAT, and clinical and research activities devoted to pleasing the admissions committees. *Your extracurriculars are for you, so do what you will enjoy doing.* Applicants often talk about their favorite extracurricular activities in their personal statements and secondary essays and during their interviews. (We discuss how to do this in the respective chapters on personal statements, secondaries, and the interview). If you sign up for activities that you don't really enjoy, you'll miss out on being able to speak passionately about your extracurriculars during these key parts of the application process.

2.2.4 Research

Research is a more important component of the application for MD-PhD applicants. If you are applying to be a 'MuD-PhuD,' you should get started with your research early in your college career. The catch-22 is, Who knows what they want to research freshman year? Here's a tip: *what* you research isn't nearly as important as *how far* you go in your research. Getting published is the ideal for PhD candidates, but group poster presentations or published abstracts are okay if you show a commitment and forward progress in whatever you choose to research. However, if you're academically strong and particularly well-rounded without any publications, you will still be a strong candidate for top MD/PhD programs. As these positions are normally fully funded, though, (they pay for your MD as well!) the onus will be on you to demonstrate your interest in and commitment to a career that involves research and clinical practice. If you emphasize one more than the other, you risk being counseled into pursuing either an MD or a PhD by itself; don't let your hard work go to waste!

To get started, you will want to search out professors on your campus who are prolific, or at least spend a majority of their time on their research. Then you just have to convince them to let you work for them, which usually isn't hard as most people don't show interest in basic science research, or offer to work for free! The only times this may be difficult is when you have a lot of premeds and few professors. In a situation like that, or in one in which you are encountering difficulty in finding a potential mentor, it's best to target younger faculty. They are usually far more motivated to take on potential mentees and are usually more inclined to create projects for interested students or allow them to pursue their interests, as long as they are somewhat in line with the laboratory's overall focus. Another perk of doing research: you'll have a strong letter of recommendation from a scientist who really knows your work (particularly if you're a non-science major)!

For non-PhD candidates, research is something in which you should have some experience, but it certainly doesn't need to be one of the main features of your application. Medical schools will want to see evidence of your familiarity with the research process. The purpose of your undergraduate research is to experience the scientific process firsthand. You want to get a feel for what it takes to engage in research and to develop a critical acumen for evaluating research. Doctors have to update their clinical practice constantly based on the latest research advances, so it's important to be able to ascertain which research studies will change the way you practice and which ones require further investigation. It helps to be familiar with different study designs (e.g. case studies, pharmaceutical trials, randomized double-blind control trials, etc.). In your required statistics class, you'll learn a bit more about evaluating the significance of study results, which will help when you're being 'pimped' on the wards at 6am. It is advantageous to be comfortable with journal articles before getting swamped in medical school!

Having said that, you can also conduct your research experience in non-hardcore science subjects, like communications, psychology, sociology, etc. The key is that the research follows the scientific process: design a study, collect data, analyze findings, and communicate results and impact. The truth is that you're not really going to ever use those basic lab techniques in medical school (except for pathology and gynecology, both of which require only the use of a microscope). So don't stress out if you normally have palpitations when someone says, "What molarity of solution ..."

By the way, for non-PhD applicants, getting published in any field is a plus, so social sciences count. If you are passionate about social-science research, it's often easier to publish in this area. 'MuD-PhuDs' need basic science research, period. Then again, if you didn't like basic lab research, you wouldn't apply for the PhD.

2.2.5   Clinical Experience

Okay, so you want to help people, right? Most everyone would answer "yes" if you asked them if they would like their career to help others. However, you can be a teacher, a firefighter, a garbage collector, etc. and make valuable contributions to society. So why choose to accomplish this as a doctor? The only answers that make sense are that you also want to make lots of money as a specialist or that you simply love the practice of medicine. Most are uncomfortable admitting that they are going into medicine for the money, and it's definitely taboo to communicate this during the application process. So you either love the practice of medicine or you need to appear to. How are you going to convince an admissions committee that you know what you are getting into and that you still love it enough to devote at least the next seven years of your life to it (four years of medical school and three years for the shortest residency)? With your clinical experience, that's how.

Most medical students volunteer with a local hospital or medical center. Many others shadow a physician in a specialty they are interested in. A few get formal jobs in a physician practice, sometimes even in administration. No medical school is expecting you to have performed brain surgery before matriculating. The key factors schools are evaluating in your clinical experience are the *longevity* of your commitment and the *settings* you chose. For example, if you are pitching yourself as a flag bearer for the uninsured, it will look good if you volunteered in a free clinic for two years.

It's pretty obvious that being premed keeps you busy. Most students wonder how they are supposed to fit clinical experience into their busy schedules. The key is to take small doses spread out over a long time. If you happen to spend your summers as an EMT, great! However, if you are the average med student, you end up squeezing in two weeks here and there with doctors who are friends of your parents. It looks better if you go once a week for fourteen weeks than if you go every day for two weeks. It's the same amount of time, but med schools want to see commitment over time. Note that the emphasis is on the duration of the experience, not the frequency. You can still accept short-term gigs if they are all you manage to arrange, or if they are important to you. For example, if you have the opportunity to volunteer in a remote village for two weeks and this really grabs you, by all means, take it. This pointer is meant to help you strategically plan your time devoted to clinical experience. Shadowing a doctor once a week instead of three times a week may be easier on the doctor, too.

We suggest that you take advantage of this opportunity to feel out what may be the rest of your life. So think about what types of medicine you can envision yourself practicing and maybe narrow that list down to your top five. Let's say you think pediatrics would be cool because you like playing with kids. Well, it would definitely behoove you to have worked in a pediatric clinic where the crying and the line of snotty-nosed, inconsolable kids waiting to see you are endless. You'll learn whether this is a field you really could love being in, and admissions committees love seeing that you have explored your interest.

Similarly, let's say you are a neuroscience major and think that you may be interested in neurology. The practice of neurology couldn't be more different than the study of neuroscience; while neuroscience explores the mind-body conundrum, is one of the most fast-paced, cutting-edge fields, and boldly bridges social and basic sciences, neurology is fraught with ambiguous diagnoses and very limited therapeutic approaches. You won't have a good sense of whether a certain field may meet your expectations unless you spend some time in the field. This will also help you down the road—most medical students are still unsure of their choice when applying to residency because they really don't have enough time to get 'the feel' of a specialty. Medical school does provide the opportunity during your clinical rotations to get experience in the basic specialty areas. However, as a medical student you are trying hard to keep up with study-ing, 'getting pimped,' and fulfilling your clinical duties during your rotations. Your undergraduate clinical experience is not burdened in this way and thus it is a better time to evaluate whether you fit in with 'the vibe' of a specialty. It may sound a bit touchy-feely, but the truth is that each specialty does have its own vibe and for that reason attracts certain types of people; for example, emergency medicine will attract distinct types of medical students from obstetrics or psychiatry.

If you are just starting college, we recommend checking them out your few top areas of interest over the next three years. If you are a second-semester junior who doesn't feel like you've really checked out what you are interested in, it's still worth get-ting some clinical experience in before the fall deadlines. Take your top choice and check it out for a few hours a week (even in one shot) during the summer—your personal statement and in-terview may actually be strongly enhanced by this experience.

So where can you get clinical experience? Anywhere! Most hos-pitals have volunteer programs and many will actually try to place you in the department of your choice if you explain that you are a premed interested in that field. Really, you could con-tact the office of any group practice and explain your interest. Find out which doctors work on which days, and then approach the one that is working when you think you can volunteer. Few doctors would say 'no' to a nice letter explaining your interest and asking if you could unobtrusively shadow them for a few hours a week. It's even better if you throw in a little bit about your background, why you are interested in the specialty, and how you really want to learn from the best.

You should tailor your experience to the type of setting you en-vision yourself working in. If you think you will be in a jungle clinic in Asia, some clinical experience abroad, or in multicul-tural settings, will be helpful. If you are going to take over your family's private practice, then working in a hospital may not be as useful as working in a private-office setting. Community clinics, hospitals, group practices, and private MD offices are all very different settings. If you are unsure of whether you would like to practice in a private or public setting, it may be a good idea to try both.

In summary, aim for clinical experience that is going to shed light on what it's like to be in the setting you think you may end up in. Remember, this is for you, not for an admissions commit-tee. You will be a stronger overall applicant if you have a good sense of what you are getting into.

2.3 Non-traditional Applicants

All your undergrad courses will count! No matter how amazing your life path was after college you will still have your GPA following you. Your pre-med prerequisites, whether they were taken in undergrad or in a post-baccalaureate program, will still be an important part of the academic portion of the application. If your science grades are weak and you're not enrolling in a postbac, we recommend considering a science-heavy master's degree program (and getting good grades in it). This will demonstrate your commitment to the profession and that you are able to handle the rigors of medical school's science curriculum.

Post-bac programs are usually associated with larger universities, but they can vary wildly. Some are highly competitive (these tend to be programs with 'special arrangements' allowing students guaranteed, binding entry into an affiliated medical school), and others allow open registration. Some post-bac programs will send their students into classes with undergraduates, while others will have specific postbac sections (which tends to happen in programs with larger enrollments). However, if schools place postbacs with undergraduates, they normally grade them on a separate curve, grading the post-bacs downward, though some programs compensate for this by setting the mean slightly higher. You should research prospective programs carefully, as there is a wide array of programs out there labelled 'postbac.'

Special master's degree programs—ones that simulate the first year of the medical school basic science curriculum—are available at select medical schools. Applicants considering these programs may have long ago taken pre-med prerequisites in which they performed well, or in which they did not perform so poorly as to warrant retaking the requirements outright (2.9–3.3 science GPA). These students are in a position to demonstrate to medical schools their handle on rigorous scientific coursework outside of a postbac. These programs sometimes allow students to take classes alongside first-year medical students, and a few even allow students who elect to choose the same school as their medical school to enter with advanced standing.

If you've been out of the academic setting for a while, other advantages of enrolling in a post-bac or a master's program include an environment of like-minded students in a similar predicament and the ability to obtain a meaningful current academic letter of recommendation. Medical schools will want an academic letter of recommendation that is a reflection of your current abilities, and they tend not to value employer feedback as highly.

Although experience in a staff setting will afford you many advantages in medical-school, admissions place more value on assessments by professors.

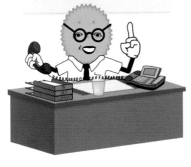

CHAPTER 3

PRIMARY APPLICATION

3.1 SIGNIFICANCE

The primary application is perhaps the most unpleasant part of the process. It requires mundane details of the past four years of your life, and, simply stated, is a pain to get through. The good news is that you don't have to think much. However, deciding which extracurricular activities merit mention, and what to say about them, may require some brain power. The most involved part of the primary, the personal statement, will be addressed in the next chapter. We'll guide you through the rest in this chapter.

When you finish, print out a copy!

The new AMCAS primary application has evolved into 18 (yup, you read that correctly, 18) mini-statements about extracurricular activities, disadvantaged status, and any institutional action/negative circumstances. These essays present a new dilemma for applicants; it's great to be able to have additional room to write about the things you've done, but figuring out what and how much to write can be overwhelming! Medical schools expect each of the appropriate essay fields to be completed. Let's start with an overview of all the fields in the application and then work on tackling the mini-statements.

3.2 Identifying Information

These fields are pretty much what they say they are—straight-forward questions about your background. They should be answered completely and honestly. Questions deal with information such as your name, contact info, schools attended, previous allopathic school matriculation, etc. You'll need to provide some rarely used info—for example, what U.S. county you were born in—as well, so make sure you can retrieve that in a timely fashion. It's a time-consuming process only because it requires such a breadth of information about you, and in considerable detail. For this reason, if you have the following in hand when starting the application, it will go much faster:

- All of your post-secondary transcripts
- You social security number
- Your resume or at least your clinical and research-related work history
- A chronological list of all your extracurricular activities
- A sugar fix and some good music!

3.2.1 Disadvantaged Status

In the Biographical Fields section, you will be presented with the question of whether or not you would like to consider yourself a disadvantaged applicant. If you reply in the affirmative, you will have to answer an essay question. According to the AMCAS, it appears that this status is largely self-designated with some loose guidelines: either you or your immediate family is poor or lives in a medically underserved area. Below is the AMCAS list of definitions to help guide your decision. Some students have gone through particularly tough circumstances in their lives, which made applying to medical school even more difficult. In the box below (Figure 3.2.1) is an example of one student's background that she considered disadvantaged but that didn't fall within the traditional guidelines. Feel free to be dramatic, but don't turn the death of your rabbit into the Odyssey.

Underserved

Do you believe, based on your own experiences or the experiences of family and friends, that the area in which you grew up was adequately served by the available health care professionals? Were there enough physicians, nurses, hospitals, clinics, and other health-care service providers?

Immediate Family

The federal government broadly defines "immediate family" as "spouse, parent, child, sibling, mother- or father-in-law, son- or daughter-in-law, or sister- or brother-in-law, including step and adoptive relationships."

State and Federal Assistance Programs

These programs are specifically defined as "Means-Tested Programs" in which the individual, family, or household income and assets must be below specified thresholds. The sponsoring agencies then provide cash and non-cash assistance to eligible individuals, families, or households. Such programs include welfare-benefit programs (federal, state, and local); Aid to Families with Dependent Children (AFDC or ADC); unemployment compensation; General Assistance (GA); food stamps; Supplemental Security Income (SSI); Medicaid; housing assistance; or other federal, state, or local financial assistance programs.

As the oldest child of Chinese immigrants, I witnessed first hand the great opportunity in the United States that everyone abroad speaks of. Going through the trials and tribulations of acculturation in the United States was how I came to realize my Chinese family dynamic was atypical. My parents, unfortunately, were typically Chinese: my father the power-hungry authoricrat, and my mother the silent and subservient buffer to his temperament. They had an arranged marriage. My mom was engaged at 16, married and living in a new country (the US) at 18, and had me at 21. Without a college degree or any vocational skills, she worked at a pancake house until I was born. Then she stayed at home to raise her first child.

My earliest memories of our family are of my mom and I driving from the police station to a domestic violence shelter. I was five. She was pregnant with my little sister and had a bloody lip. We had nowhere to go. She couldn't afford for us to live alone, and we couldn't stay at the shelter for more than a week. Chinese society doesn't support divorce (especially back then), and Chinese social standards tell women they should treat their husbands as gods. Men are infallible and women powerless. Even many of her friends were suffering silently with alcoholic or abusive husbands.

Ironically, one of the best events for my family was the first time my father went to prison. I was in fourth grade. At first my mom took us back to China. She quickly realized that was not the best option for her children (education, opportunity), and that she was an outcaste as a single mother. She returned to the US with resolve to take advantage of US education and opportunity herself. We lived in an apartment over the office she was working in. She went to night school and got a degree in business administration. I watched my little sister and packed our lunches. A year later she sent my sister and me to California, where she thought we would do better. For six months we stayed with distant family friends whom we had never met. My sister was in first grade and cried every night. We were tired of moving and starting over, but we grew stronger in our love and support for each other.

Two years later, my father came out of prison—supposedly reformed. My mom took him back. We didn't really know him, and it was hard to adjust to his wanting to control our lives again. He stayed sober for a few years, but then fell into his old patterns. We all danced around his moods and demands. My mom worked nights and we dreaded being alone with him, never knowing if he was going to be drunk; sometimes emotional and effusive, sometimes criticizing. School was the only escape. I held on to my education with my life. I earned a scholarship to a private high school and worked in the school cafeteria to pay my way.

Fortunately, my mother evolved in her role and made a decision that was unorthodox to her native culture—she spoke out against my father and divulged the 25 years of his physical and emotional abuse. My father's response was to abandon us. For the last ten years, we have been unaware of his whereabouts. We were abandoned by Chinese society as well: rumors spread that my mom was so terrible that she made my father leave. Despite this, my mother rose to the challenge of raising two daughters and managing a household with amazing grace. Ostensibly, from her I have learned to value my independence and to believe in my capabilities.

Through scholarships, grants, and student loans, I have been blessed with the opportunity to obtain a great education. Throughout college, and even today I've worked to help support my mother and sister. We work together as a family to meet our needs. Every penny counts.

Designating yourself as disadvantaged is not based solely on economic circumstances, nor is it based on ethnicity. For example, an applicant living in a well-off household that was a ninety-minute drive from the nearest secondary- or tertiary-care center could self-designate as disadvantaged. You might think that such a scenario couldn't occur, but it does. Based on the AMCAS questions, this applicant could be considered disadvantaged. Medical schools are obligated to increase the diversity of their entering classes by making efforts to include both underrepresented minorities and those that lived in underserved areas, with the rationale that the latter group wwill eventually return to their homes and help alleviate that area's shortage of medical professionals.

Other information you may need in order to answer the disadvantaged questions include whether or not your family received state or federal assistance, their income level (if you do not know or don't want to answer, that is okay), and what resources you used to pay for your post-secondary schooling (not exact numbers but percentage estimates). Following this, you'll have an opportunity to write a mini-statement about why you feel you are disadvantaged.

Even though the disadvantaged mini-statement is optional, everyone who believes him or herself to be disadvantaged should write this mini-statement. It will greatly increase your probability of receiving this designation. In addition, many medical schools will use this mini-statement to consider you for disadvantaged-student scholarships. This mini-statement is similar to the personal statement in that it is your chance to speak your mind and let the committee get to know you; the two statements may even be used to complement one another. A few students choose to write their personal statement on their growth and experience getting through a tough time, and then use the same essay for the disadvantaged mini-statement.

Figure 3.2.1 Sample Disadvantaged Mini-Statement

3.2.2   Institutional Action

This section applies to applicants who are on academic probation or conduct violation. If this applies to you, make sure you take the time to explain in the mini-statement space provided. If a medical school is going to accept someone who has institutional action on their record, they need to feel good about. Schools appreciate honesty, remorse, and growth. It's better to say that you realize how immature you were, that you faced the consequences, and that you truly learned your lesson, than to make yourself seem like a victim.

3.3 DESIGNATING COURSES FOR YOUR SCIENCE (BCPM DESIGNATION) GPA

Have your official or unofficial transcripts handy or this section will take forever! AMCAS is pretty specific and exhaustive (e.g. course numbers, school years and terms, class standing, course classification, and type of credit received. The AMCAS specific designations, ones that your school transcript may or may not tell you, are the course classification and the "special course types" section. For course classification, AMCAS is fairly specific, as they use the designations to determine what gets included in your all-important science GPA, an important admissions criterion for all medical schools—sometimes mores important than your overall GPA. Course classification is described in AMCAS materials as follows:

BEHAVIORAL & SOCIAL SCIENCES (BESS)
- ☐ Anthropology
- ☐ Economics
- ☐ Family Studies
- ☐ Psychology
- ☐ Sociology

BIOLOGY (BIOL) - BCPM
- ☐ Anatomy
- ☐ Biology
- ☐ Biophysics
- ☐ Biotechnology
- ☐ Botany
- ☐ Cell Biology
- ☐ Ecology
- ☐ Entomology
- ☐ Genetics
- ☐ Histology
- ☐ Immunology
- ☐ Microbiology
- ☐ Molecular Biology
- ☐ Neuroscience
- ☐ Physiology

BUSINESS (BUSI)
- ☐ Accounting
- ☐ Business
- ☐ Finance
- ☐ Human Resource Studies
- ☐ Management
- ☐ Organizational Studies
- ☐ Marketing

CHEMISTRY (CHEM) - BCPM
- ☐ Biochemistry
- ☐ Chemistry
- ☐ Physical Chemistry
- ☐ Thermodynamics

COMMUNICATIONS (COMM)
- ☐ Journalism
- ☐ Media Production & Studies
- ☐ TV, Video, & Audio

COMPUTER SCIENCE/ TECHNOLOGY (COMP)
- ☐ Computer Science
- ☐ Computer Engineering
- ☐ Information Systems
- ☐ Telecommunications

EDUCATION (EDUC)
- ☐ Counseling & Personnel Services
- ☐ Curriculum & Instruction
- ☐ Educational Policy
- ☐ Educational Administration

☐ Health Education
☐ Human Development
☐ Physical Education (except for sports courses such as tennis, golf, aerobics, etc. Use Other for these types of courses.)
☐ Special Education

Engineering (ENGI)
☐ Aerospace Engineering
☐ Biomedical Engineering
☐ Chemical Engineering
☐ Civil Engineering
☐ Electrical Engineering
☐ Engineering
☐ Environmental Engineering
☐ Mechanical Engineering
☐ Nuclear Engineering

English Language & Literature (ENGL)
☐ English Composition & Rhetoric
☐ English Creative Writing
☐ English Language & Literature

Fine Arts (ARTS)
☐ Art
☐ Art History
☐ Dance
☐ Fine Arts
☐ Music
☐ Photography
☐ Theatre

Health Sciences (HEAL)
☐ Allied Health
☐ Chiropractic
☐ Dentistry
☐ Hearing & Speech Sciences
☐ Hospital Administration

☐ Kinesiology
☐ Medical Technology
☐ Medicine
☐ Nursing
☐ Nutrition & Food Sciences
☐ Occupational Therapy
☐ Optometry

Health Sciences (HEAL) continued
☐ Osteopathy
☐ Physical Therapy
☐ Physician Assistant
☐ Public Health
☐ Pharmacology & Pharmacy
☐ Sports Medicine
☐ Veterinary Medicine

History (HIST)
☐ History
☐ Foreign Languages/ Linguistics/Lit. (FLAN)
☐ American Sign Language
☐ Comparative Literature
☐ Linguistics
☐ Foreign Language(s) & Literature

Government/Political Sci/ Law (GOVT)
☐ Criminology & Criminal Justice
☐ Government
☐ International Relations & Studies
☐ Law/Legal Studies
☐ Political Science
☐ Public Affairs & Policy
☐ Urban Policy & Planning

Math (MATH) - BCPM
☐ Applied Mathematics
☐ Mathematics
☐ Statistics

Natural/Physical Sciences (NPSC)
☐ Agriculture
☐ Animal and Avian Sciences
☐ Forestry
☐ Geography
☐ Geology
☐ Horticulture
☐ Landscape Architecture
☐ Meteorology
☐ Natural Resources
☐ Oceanography
☐ Environmental Science & Policy

Other (OTHR)
All courses which do not fit appropriately into another category, including:
☐ Architecture
☐ Interdisciplinary courses
☐ Library Science
☐ Military Science
☐ Sports (tennis, golf, aerobics, etc.)

Philosophy/Religion (PHIL)
☐ Ethics
☐ Logic
☐ Philosophy
☐ Religion
☐ Theology

Physics (PHYS) - BCPM
☐ Astronomy
☐ Physics

Special Studies (SSTU)
☐ Afro-American Studies
☐ American Studies
☐ Gender Studies

The BCPM suffix is used to denote classifications included in the BCPM (science) GPA calculation. These guidelines are meant to help you sort out courses that may be taught in different departments than transcripts indicate; for example, a biopsychology course taught by your school's psychology department can be classified as biology and included in BCPM. However, if AMCAS disagrees with your self-classification, it can mean lengthy delays in verification and recalculation of your GPA. As a result, you should ensure that you have syllabi handy, or a good course catalog description, to justify your classification to AMCAS should your application hit a snag.

3.4 WORK AND ACTIVITIES

This is probably by far the most time-consuming part of the primary application. The recent limitation to 15 "activities" overall—this includes anything from extracurriculars to awards and honors to work experience—and the addition of the 15 mini-statements have made this section a bit more challenging. However, like every section of free prose on the application, these mini-statements are another way to differentiate yourself from other applicants. In many cases, a lot of the information you may want to use for your personal statement will overlap with information you'll want to include here. If you're going to expand on something in your personal statement, you don't need to expand on it in your mini-statements, and vice versa. If you must talk about the same activity in these two parts of the primary application, the key is to highlight different facets of the experience in each section. Save your choice experiences for your personal statement (as you will see in the next chapter), and write about the other good ones here. Don't feel that you have to write something for every experience you list—the more overwhelming it looks, the less likely it is to be read. Don't forget, admissions committees already have to review your GPA, MCAT score, and personal statement before they focus on extracurricular activities. Your extracurricular activities are important, but more so for *what* you did than for how you describe them here. Another place you will be asked to elaborate on your experiences will be during your interviews, which is the most important discussion of them. Some secondary essays may also ask you to delve into these, so rest assured they will get some attention and your efforts over the last four years will not have been in vain.

That being said, here are some more concrete tips directly from admissions directors of a few ivy-league medical schools:

"We advise applicants to use the work/activities section to provide clarifying or descriptive information, not to write mini-essays."

"They should briefly describe the activity and not assume all readers know what it was. They want to let the reader know why/how the activity was significant enough to list, and they should do this by including something that says what they gained from it and/or contributed by doing it. I tell them not to assume the reader will know the significance or usefulness of any activity. They supply that. Keep it brief; med schools like that. Since the personal statement should not be a list of activities in narrative form, a number, perhaps most or all of the activities, may not have been mentioned in the essay they wrote."

"Write only about particularly meaningful activities, and only those which you did not discuss in the personal statement. It's okay not to fill all 15 spaces, especially if you are dedicated to only a few activities."

Simply stated:

- Don't inundate your application. Only write something if the information you provide is truly adding value.

- Don't succumb to the temptation to fill every box immediately! Take a step back to organize your thoughts about your activities. Order is not important as medical schools can change the order after you've submitted.

- Keep your personal statement and your mini-statements distinct. Use the mini-statements as a space to highlight what you did not address in your personal statement.

- If you have more than 15 activities or honors that you want medical schools to know about, consider grouping them into time or topical categories. For example, you could include all your activities from one summer under one entry, or all snorkeling tours you led over your summers in Oceania under one entry. If you have fewer than 15, no worries; medical schools would rather you be dedicated to a few activities rather than dabble in many.

"If you write your personal statement on why bowling opened your eyes to the beauty and spirituality surrounding plastic surgery, center your mini-statements on other activities and only include basic details of bowling (e.g. responsibilities, length of involvement, etc.) in the mini-statement section.

- **This is the only section in which to list your awards and honors**. If you have them, save one of your 15 boxes and enter Awards/Honors and then list them with the dates in the description space.

Example of a good and succinct activity description:

> **Tutoring**
>
> French: I tutored two struggling Native-American students twice a week. I was able to help them get their first passing grades in a foreign language.
>
> Math: I tutored through Upward Bound, an organization linking area students with disadvantaged high school students, three times a week during the summer.

*Example of '**doing too much**' in an activity description:*

> **Library Administrative Assistant**
>
> Worked 10 hours/week at Olin Chemistry Library at Cornell. It was an exhilarating experience; during down times, I spent hours browsing the organic chemistry literature. Life is a constant learning experience, and I knew that mastering organic chemistry, at whatever cost, was paramount. *Meso* compounds had this innate beauty about them that I rarely encountered, even in the art museums of Paris and Vienna. This experience solidified my decision to pursue medicine; interacting with an eminent scientific community four times a week in Cornell's hallowed chemistry department inspired me to do chemistry research as well.

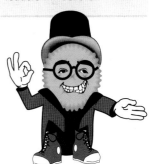

Meso compounds? At least pick something I... err, your readers will believe.

3.5 LETTERS OF RECOMMENDATION

3.5.1 Who to Ask

Many applicants feel they need to have recommendations from science teachers and doctors alone. This is untrue! The other common misconception is that the more letters you have, the better. It is best to restrict your recommendation-gathering to professors and research/activity mentors with whom you've had a close working relationship. Simply stated, people who know you better will write better letters. Plus, it can be easy to get bogged down in the mundane process of obtaining recommendation letters, committee letters, and waivers. It's unfortunately commonplace to have to encourage recommenders to make deadlines, so it's better to pick people who are excited about supporting your application.

Medical schools value letters written by people who have had the opportunity to observe you over an extended period of time and evaluate your performance. A professor with whom you earned high marks (A, A–, B+) is a good choice, as is a work or volunteer supervisor who has consistently given you solid evaluations.

You should aim for at least one letter from a science professor, since his or her assessment will help medical schools to gauge your ability to withstand the rigors of the medical school curriculum. Asking a professor in your major subject is also helpful, as medical schools will want an assessment of your performance in your chosen field of study. Lastly, people who have mentored you in your extracurricular activities, whether the osteopath you shadowed or your basketball coach, are considered important recommenders. Asking deans, family, friends, your family physician, your life coach, or other individuals who are unlikely to be able to provide medical schools with an evaluation of your intellectual capabilities is not helpful to your application, and may even leave medical schools questioning your judgment.

3.5.2 Making the Request

Be respectful by making sure you give your recommenders plenty of time to write your letter, as it is likely many other students have approached them with similar requests. Three weeks is a reasonable guideline, though your recommenders will probably be appreciative if you give them even more time. In general, the earlier you ask, the more likely they are to oblige. If you are graduating soon but want to apply within the next few years, you should determine whether your school can store your letters of recommendation with the school/premed committee or a credentials service. This way, your professors will have the opportunity to write about you with fresh memories, and you've saved yourself the work of having to get back in touch later. If you're already a few years out, don't worry too much; though you may not expect it, professors often remember their students well for many years, particularly in smaller or more advanced courses.

Before approaching professors, you should organize some paperwork to help them get a sense of your accomplishments and your career goals and aspirations. A professor can write a much stronger letter about you if he or she has a copy of your resume (if you don't yet have one, make one!), and at least a preliminary personal statement addressing the first two Cardinal Questions (refer to **Glossary** or **Chapter 4: Your Personal Statement** for definition and tips on getting started). With this information, the professor can tie his or her assessment of you in the course/laboratory to your career goals in a positive and synergistic way. Don't sell yourself short by simply handing your writers a recommendation-request form; give them all the tools they might need to be more effective cheerleaders for you.

Once you've decided who to ask, and have a resume and personal statement to present to them, you'll need to sort out some logistical issues that will arise. First of all, you will need to decide whether you want to waive your right to view the letter of recommendation, a right to which you are entitled by the Family Educational Rights & Privacy Act of 1974. It is generally thought that medical schools weigh confidential letters more heavily as they are seen as more candid assessments. Therefore, it's best to ask writers you are confident will say positive things, so that you can sign the waiver *before* you hand them the forms. If you have any doubts or concerns about what a writer will say, this is a good sign that you should ask somebody else.

3.6 RESEARCHING SCHOOLS I (SELECTING RECIPIENT SCHOOLS)

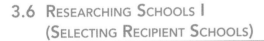

At this point, your research is focused on determining not only where you may potentially want to go (dream or reality), but also where your 'numbers' fall in line with medical schools' admitted classes. Applying to 10 schools is realistic, and up to 20 is common. At this stage in the process you'll want to look at the average accepted student's profile and see how you compare. We recommend always going to the school website directly for the most up-to-date information. Almost all schools provide a profile of their most recent accepted class. (If it's not on their website, they will usually provide you with this information if you ask for it.) If you don't know where to start, AAMC will provide you with a complete list of all medical schools, and they also give the latest information on GPAs and MCAT scores for all applicants any given year. They provide this information for free and even organize it according to state, gender, and a few other variables.

Ideally, you'll apply to a few schools for which you match their average accepted student profile, a few for which you are just below the average numbers, and at least one or two schools for which your numbers are stronger than their average applicants. In this manner, you'll have a 'backup' school or two, a realistic

Remember that average values mean that values both above and below have been included. An accepted class with an average GPA of 3.5 includes students that may have had a 3.3, as well as a few with a 3.7. So, don't be totally discouraged if you are a bit below the average numbers. If you are really interested in the school, you should still apply. Just make sure your personal statement is strong!

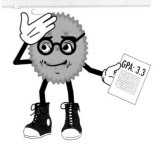

chance of getting into schools you are interested in, and a chance at your 'pie-in-the-sky' schools. You'll want to think about what factors are really important to you in choosing a school. Some applicants must live in a certain location, and so they will want to research only schools in their area. Others may be after a joint degree and will want to make their selection based on this criterion. So, in short, reflect on which schools you think you may be interested in, check out the profile of their average accepted student and strategically narrow down your list to schools whose profiles you match, including one 'backup' and one 'pie-in-the-sky' school.

---

www.aamc.org/data/facts

www.usnews.com

http://en.wikipedia.org/wiki/University_ranking

http://grants2.nih.gov/grants/award/trends/medschc.htm

http://services.aamc.org/currdir/section2/start.cfm
(joint degree)

Table of Online Resources

3.7 MD/PhD APPLICANTS

In addition to the "Personal Comments" essay, you will need to write a MD/PhD statement and a "Significant Research Experience" essay. MD/PhD committees are interested in the following points:

- **Solid research experiences**—You should have experience conducting research projects that resulted in a publication, abstract, presentation at a scientific conference, or important results. You need to demonstrate to these committees that you're familiar with the world of research and have taken advantage of research opportunities.

- **Exposure to clinical medicine**—You need to show MD/PhD committees that you're not simply a research junkie who spurns patient interaction. The burden of proof rests upon your ability to persuade these committees why neither a MD nor PhD alone will suffice in fulfilling your career goals.

Additional tips:

- You should provide a brief introduction into the field and topic of your prior research.

- It behooves you to select research that is related to the type of research you wish to pursue in the MD/PhD program. If your research is unrelated, make sure you address why you have decided to make this change.

The Personal Statement

4.1 Before You Begin...

4.1.1 Purpose of the Personal Statement

The personal statement is a vital component to your AMCAS application. Above all else, your statement is *your way of securing an interview*. The fixed parts of your application—grades, recommendations, MCAT scores (hopefully Examkrackers helped you feel good about this!)—hold a lot of weight, but most top applicants will have similar grades, scores, and experiences. Think of the personal statement as your opportunity to differentiate yourself from the pack. Unlike other parts of the application the personal statement is a chance to actually show your personality. This chapter will help you prepare to demonstrate why you are a unique and genuine person.

Yes, we know the personal statement is daunting! However, you've already written one to be admitted into your current undergraduate institution. The purpose of this personal statement is no different. It's about showing maturity and growth from your past experiences, and your potential for continued growth. However, you also need to tie in your undying devotion to medicine and step up your marketing strategy.

You may be wondering, "What marketing strategy?!" Being able to market yourself is often difficult for students, usually because they lack experience doing so. You've gotten to where you are by working hard and getting good grades; now you have to sell the product of that investment. Many applicants are ruffled by this concept: "I'm going to be a doctor, not a sales rep!" But, getting into medical school has only continued to become tougher, and as in any scenario where demand exceeds supply, the cost of getting in has gone up. If you want to get accepted to a U.S. medical institution, especially one of the top ones, you have to be willing to go the extra mile. The good news is that you have already been doing this (e.g. taking organic chemistry and physics, taking the MCAT instead of the GRE) just to have gotten this far. The other good news is that we are going to guide you through the process.

The personal statement is your thirty-second Superbowl ad. Air time isn't easy to come by, but it's high-yield for making an impression. It is crucial that you market your selling points quickly and concisely, grab and keep the reader's attention, and leave him or her wanting more. You're fighting for the reader's time, which is at a premium; if the person is not hooked, he or she has hundreds of other applicant folders to move on to. After reading your essay, the reader should feel like he or she knows you, and likes you (or at least respects you enough to think you will be a fine candidate and future physician). You've spent a lot of money, time, and energy building your success in school, so it's important to spend time optimizing your personal statement. Keep these points in mind as you're brainstorming ideas and composing the statement; it will help you stay motivated. The personal statement takes time, energy, creativity, and guts. A solid personal statement is the foundation of a winning self-marketing strategy.

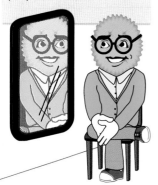

"I'm good enough. I'm smart enough. And gosh darn it, people like me!"

4.2 Our 'Five Golden Steps' to Conquering the Personal Statement

4.2.1 Step 1: The First 2 'Cardinal Questions'

You probably have experiences and achievements that make you stand out from your peers. That's great! For the personal statement, you want to focus on ideas that help you answer these two cardinal questions. You absolutely must address these questions in your personal statement.

Why do I want to go to medical school?

Why should medical school want me?

These questions may seem obvious, but with the pressure to make yourself look as good as possible in an application, a competitive applicant can end up with a personal statement that's more of an extended brag. An even larger number of students forget to make sure that they answer both questons—too many admissions essays address only *one* of these questions. Applying to medical school is a two-way street—you need to demonstrate that you will make them look good, and also explain why you want to make this huge investment.

The best way to get started is to start brainstorming possible answers to these questions. Don't stress!—this is just for you right now. We're going to come back to this brainstorm later in Step 3. Making sure you've answered the first two cardinal questions is also an important check at the very *end* of the writing process; after many revisions, applicants often restructure their essays and forget to check! In Figure 4.2.1 below, our sample student, Cheyenne Ng Starr, brainstorms her answers to these two cardinal questions.

Why Medicine?	Why Me?
• *Healing is important to me* • *Ayurvedic-healing family background* • *Human body is the ultimate form of art to me*	• *Creative* • *Passionate* • *Approach medicine as an art* • *Approach problems from many different angles—interdisciplinary* • *Care about betterment of humankind*

Figure 4.2.1 Sample Cardinal Question Brainstorm

Following these next steps will help you present answers to these questions in a polished, coherent, and even personal manner.

4.2.2 Step 2: Constructing a Self-Reflection Chart

What Do I Write About?

Though you will need to answer the two cardinal questions, the actual *topic* of your personal statement is left completely up to you. You have creative license here! We've read successful essays on guinea pigs, caramel fudge brownies, and even haikus. The topic can be an elusive concept because the essay is really about **you**. The topic is just a *theme* that may run through the essay and help the reader to remember the applicant—"Oh, the guinea pig guy!" For this reason, we call this theme a 'gift wrap'—it's a superficial theme adorning the real present (you), and can be used to distinguish yourself. Choosing a gift wrap is our last step, for the same reason that your high school English teacher made you write your introduction and conclusion paragraphs *after* you'd written the rest of the essay. It's *what* you are writing about that is most important. *How* you present it is very important, but secondary. So let's keep focusing on you for now.

Let's Brainstorm!

If you ask anyone to tell you about themselves, their first reaction is to look startled or to stall. How do you begin to answer a question that broad? Naturally, it's one you want to answer well. A good start to telling medical schools about yourself is to consider the categories below. These are the facets of your life that they are almost uniformly interested in:

- ⊙ **Experiences**—This includes aspects of your personal life.

- ⊙ **Motivations and Goals**

- ⊙ **Inspirational Figures**—Someone that is actually in your life is always better than a landmark figure whom you didn't or don't know personally.

- ⊙ **Research**

- ⊙ **Extracurricular Interests**—Anything you spend time on that is not directly related to medicine.

- ⊙ **Personal Characteristics**—These will help you to weave your Superbowl-worthy statement together but should not be a major focus of the personal statement (unless you are a creative writing major).

No sex, drugs, or rock n roll unless it relates to urology, pharmaceutical research, or neurology.

Think about all six of these topic areas, even if you have particularly strong examples for certain ones. We've organized these topics into three columns in the chart below (**Figure 4.2.2a**): Experiences, Personal Characteristics, and Motivation. For each category, it is a good idea to jot down notes on the 'basic information' about the category and on '*lessons learned.*'

To explain further, we have included sample questions you may ask yourself as you gather your thoughts. The questions are designed to stimulate your creative thought process; by no means limit yourself to these questions. You may have to look up some information such as dates and official job titles to refresh your memory. Don't worry, not everything in the chart will be used in the essay in the long run. (Remember, you have only a page or two.) Nevertheless, having all of this information in one place is invaluable, not only for convenience, but also for gauging what is best to include in the essay.

The 'Lessons Learned' boxes are provided as a space to organize your thoughts and reactions to each of your experiences. Thinking about what lessons you have learned from your experiences, your personal growth, or inspirational figures is going to help you:

- Pick what to include in your essay (Step 3)
- Answer the first two cardinal questions (Step 1)
- Demonstrate your ability to reflect internally and analyze a situation
- Prepare for your interview (Chapter 6)

Medical schools want personal statements to go far beyond a laundry list of achievements, since they can get much of that information from other parts of your application. Admissions committees look to the personal statement for an indication of the applicant's *analytical capabilities* and his or her *facility for self-reflection and growth*.

As you fill out this chart, you may have noticed that it's very similar to the extracurricular list on the AMCAS online application. If you haven't yet tackled that part of the application, thinking about the questions in this chart will help you complete that list. If you have already filled in the extracurricular-activities list, this will still help you to complete this step; for this chart, you should *only* include what you're willing to write about and flesh out details of what you did and what you learned from it.

> These questions will help you gain greater self-awareness that will help you not only in writing the statement, but also in solidifying and clarifying your decision to study medicine, making you more competitive.

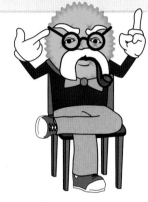

	COLUMN 1: EXPERIENCES	COLUMN 2: PERSONAL CHARACTERISTICS	COLUMN 3: MOTIVATION
	Clinical Experiences	**Strengths**	**Goals in Medicine**
Basic Information	*Where did you work, and for how long?* *What did you do?*	*What do you think are your best qualities?* *What have others said are your more admirable qualities?*	*What do you hope to achieve?* *What speciality are you interested in?*
Lessons Learned			
	Extracurricular Experiences	**Weaknesses**	**Inspirational Figures**
Basic Information	*What experiences did you have that were unique?* *Which ones make interesting conversation?*	*What obstacles, personal or external, have you faced/are facing in life?* *What about your work ethic or attitude has held you back?*	*Has anyone close to you had a significant impact on your life?* *Who was it?*
Lessons Learned			
	Research	**Quirks**	**Other Interests**
Basic Information	*Have you worked on any research (scientific or not)?* *How did you get involved?* *What was your role?* *Did you see any results?*	*Is there anything unique about you that may be interesting?*	*Have you kept up with scientific advances (or another field)?*
Lessons Learned			

Figure 4.2.2a What is a Self-Reflection Chart?

We've divided experiences into how medical schools perceive them: those that are related to medicine (research and clinical experience), and then everything else. When it comes to experiences in the latter category, however, you will still need to address why they are related to medicine for you. Experiences that are health-related include volunteer work (hospitals, clinics), field work (public health outreach, education), and research (basic science, clinical, or public health, health economics, etc.). Extracurricular experiences include any school-related activity (debate, community service, etc.), family and childhood experiences (financial difficulty, divorce, death in the family, etc.), and personal hobbies and interests to which you devoted a significant amount of time (acting, yoga, running your own business, etc.). Medical schools respond to off-beat, interesting experiences, especially if they had an impact on how you think about medicine or why you want to be a physician. If you are lucky (or unfortunate) enough to have such an experience, bring it into your writing!

In the second column, we've separated personal qualities into strengths, weaknesses, and quirks. In this column, you should reflect on your attributes. Be honest—your sincerity will show. Think of some good qualities you've demonstrated in recent years, and how they might make you a better physician. For weaknesses, the discussion is open to ones you've since overcome. Drawing attention to any persisting weaknesses will help you as much as a gallstone. Medical schools know everyone has experienced obstacles and setbacks, but they expect that you've moved beyond them. Discussing growth through a personal weakness is a great tool to demonstrate what *skills* you have used, and *insight* you have gained, in the process. So don't be afraid! Remember, medicine is becoming 'humanized'—there are enough doctors with god complexes.

The third column encompasses your 'Motivations,' which may include your goals in your medical career, people whom have inspired you, and other interests which have fuelled your passion for medicine. [Hint: "Because my parents want me to be a doctor" and "I want to make a lot of money" are not good answers.]

In the sample chart below (**Figure 4.2.2b**), you can see how Cheyenne has completed her self-reflection.

	COLUMN 1: EXPERIENCES	COLUMN 2: PERSONAL CHARACTERISTICS	COLUMN 3: MOTIVATIONS
	Clinical	**Strengths**	**Goals in Medicine**
Basic Information	• *Landmark Medical Center; Counselling Intern; Inpatient facility for schizophrenic inpatients; fall 1998* • *Amgen; Genetic counselling intern; counselled high-risk pregnancies; spring 1998* • *St. Josephs Medical Center; volunteer; helped with pediatric patients; spring 1996*	• *Multidisciplinary approach to problems* • *Teamwork/Communication* • *Leadership* • *Funny* • *Spiritual* • *Always growing & learning* • *Care about betterment of humankind* • *Passionate* • *Creative*	• *Neurology* • *Psychiatry* • *Infectious diseases* • *Public Health* • *Not sure* • *Not Research!*
Lessons Learned	• *Like counselling* • *Realized patients make decisions based on different value systems than docs*		
	Extracurricular	**Weaknesses**	**Inspirational Figures**
Basic Information	• ***Living in Italy*** • ***Art/Painting*** • *Spoken word/poetry* • *Dancing* • *International travel: India, Europe, South America* • *Collegians for Youth* • *South Asian Students Association*	• *Family! Lots of personal obstacles* • *Cultural obstacles being a first-generation woman* • *Lack of patience* • *Stubborn/lack flexibility* • *Don't like authority* • *Get bored fast*	• *Grandma—Ayurvedic healer and midwife*
Lessons Learned	• ***Art and medicine make me feel the same sense of fulfillment*** • ***Medicine is just like art to me***	• *Drawing boundaries* • *Seeking positive company (including other powerful women)* • *Communication*	• *Healing is a holistic process— must consider the whole person, not just the ailment* • *Natural approaches to healing*
	Research	**Quirks**	**Other Interests**
Basic Information	• *Mt. Sinai Medical Center; Volunteer Lab Assistant; studying Hyaluronidase cancer markers; summer 2000*	• *Many languages* • *Great bartender*	• ***Neuroscience major*** • *Viral oncogenesis* • *HIV/AIDS*
Lessons Learned	• *Don't like lab setting! Prefer working with patients/human interaction*	• *Appreciate different cultures* • *Appreciate a good drink!* • *Learned that people always want someone to talk to*	• *May relate to my specialty in future?* • ***Amazed at how unique we are in brain function/ personality...works of art!*** • *Amazed by the power of both nature and nurture on personal development*

Figure 4.2.2b Sample Completed Self-Reflection Chart

4.2.3   Step 3: Connecting the Dots

Now, you have a completed chart displaying your experiences and the qualities you exhibited in or acquired from each one. To create the body of your personal statement,

1. **Pick one or two of your experiences from Column 1 that you would like to write about.** Limiting yourself to one or two experiences will help you focus, allowing you to write about one topic in depth rather than overloading your statement with rushed explanations of multiple experiences.

   or

   Pick one or two of your motivations from Column 3 that you would like to write about. Your goals and interests are just as important as your experiences. Applicants are often so busy worrying about proving that they are worthy based on their experiences that they forget this. You do not have to base your whole essay on your clinical background! Remember, your AMCAS application provides admissions committees with a list of all your experiences, and even allows some space to describe them. Oftentimes, essays that focus on your passions and ambitions are easier to write and more interesting to read!

   You can do both! Just because you have chosen to write about your motivations doesn't mean that you can't mention an experience that is relevant. Similarly, it is often really easy to tie in your motivations while writing about your experiences. Keep in mind, however, that you have limited space and don't want the essay to be too crammed. Alternatively, you may choose to talk about one topic from your Experiences Column and one from your Motivations (as in Cheyenne's Sample Essay).

2. **Pick which of your qualities from Column 2 you can demonstrate while you write about the experiences or motivations you have chosen.**

3. **When picking which topics to write about, refer back to your brainstorm on the two cardinal questions.** Remember, it is through your discussion of your experiences and motivations that you answer the first of the cardinal questions, why you want to go into medicine. It is through the lessons you have learned, or the qualities you demonstrated in your experiences or motivations, that you answer the second cardinal question, why you are going to be a great doctor.

Cheyenne chose to focus her essay on one topic from her motivations (in blue text in **Figures 4.2.3a & 4.2.3b**) and one from her experiences (**Figures 4.2.3a & 4.2.3b**, in red text). She chooses to discuss some of the lessons she has learned from these topics. Then, she picks personal characteristics to describe in her discussion of these topics. Notice how her topic choice is influenced by her brainstorm for answering the two cardinal questions (**Figure 4.2.1**). Here is her Connect-the-Dots:

> - (**Motivation**) Neuroscience major → (**Lessons Learned**) humans are unique works of art → (**Strengths**) multidisciplinary & comprehensive approach to problems, good with teamwork
>
> - (**Extracurricular Experience**) Living in Italy/Painting → (**Lessons Learned**) Medicine and art both give me the same sense of fulfillment → (**Strengths**) renewal of self/constantly growing & learning while healing others and serving betterment of humankind; (**Weaknesses**) lack of flexibility—appreciate how things are constantly changing in medicine

Figure 4.2.3a Sample Connect-the-dots

Cheyenne Ng Starr included the items highlighted in green below (**Figure 4.2.3b**) in her essay (**Figure 4.2.5b**). There is a lot she did not include and that is good. Many of the items that she just mentioned she did not pick out initially but found an opportunity to throw in while she was writing. These items are also highlighted in green in her essay (**Figure 4.2.5b**).

COLUMN 1: EXPERIENCES	COLUMN 2: PERSONAL CHARACTERISTICS	COLUMN 3: MOTIVATIONS
Clinical	**Strengths**	**Goals in Medicine**
Basic Information • Landmark Medical Center; Counselling Intern; Inpatient facility for schizophrenic inpatients; fall 1998 • Amgen; Genetic counselling intern; counselled high-risk pregnancies; spring 1998 • St. Josephs Medical Center; volunteer; helped with pediatric patients; spring 1996	• Multidisciplinary approach to problems • Teamwork/Communication • Leadership • Funny • Spiritual • Always growing & learning • Care about betterment of humankind • Passionate • Creative	• Neurology • Psychiatry • Infectious diseases • Public Health • Not sure • Not Research!
Lessons Learned • Like counselling • Realized patients make decisions based on different value systems than docs		
Extracurricular	**Weaknesses**	**Inspirational Figures**
Basic Information • Living in Italy • Art/Painting • Spoken word/poetry • Dancing • International travel: India, Europe, South America • Collegians for Youth • South Asian Students Association	• Family! Lots of personal obstacles • Cultural obstacles being a first-generation woman • Lack of patience • Stubborn/lack flexibility • Don't like authority • Get bored fast	• Grandma—Ayurvedic healer and midwife
Lessons Learned • Art and medicine make me feel the same sense of fulfillment • Medicine is just like art to me	• Drawing boundaries • Seeking positive company (including other powerful women) • Communication	• Healing is a holistic process—must consider the whole person, not just the ailment • Natural approaches to healing
Research	**Quirks**	**Other Interests**
Basic Information • Mt. Sinai Medical Center; Volunteer Lab Assistant; studying Hyaluronidase cancer markers; summer 2000	• Many languages • Great bartender	• Neuroscience major • Viral oncogenesis • HIV/AIDS
Lessons Learned • Don't like lab setting! Prefer working with patients/human interaction	• Appreciate different cultures • Appreciate a good drink! • Learned that people always want someone to talk to	• May relate to my specialty in future? • Amazed at how unique we are in brain function/personality...works of art! • Amazed by the power of both nature and nurture on personal development

Figure 4.2.3b Sample Self-Reflection Chart with Selected Topics & Connect-the-dots

4.2.4   Step 4: Choose Your 'Gift Wrap'

For the best selection, you're going to want to hit Bloomingdale's on 59th and 3rd... just kidding. Picking your gift wrap—the theme you want to surround your essay's body—is a key way to stand out from 99% of medical school applicants. If chosen well, your gift wrap will grab the reader's interest, create a connection to your experience that your reader can relate to, and provide material for a brief analysis in the conclusion of your essay. Your gift wrap is your personal stamp, so bring your personality and flair into your choice. It will make your essay stand out, and perhaps make it a subject of admissions office chatter and the reason you will stick in an interviewer's mind (we're speaking from experience here!). It's also a great way to sneak another aspect of your personality into the statement. Confused? Look below for some examples that were used successfully—the gift wrap and its accompanying body—to clarify what you will need to incorporate into your gift wrap and how it needs to function.

When choosing your gift wrap, just remember it's not the meat of the essay—it just adds a little bit of flavor to your answers to the cardinal questions! For this reason, the gift wrap is usually only present in the introduction and conclusion paragraphs. Others may choose to carry their theme, or gift wrap, throughout the essay. Below are examples of gift wrap in two successful personal statements; as you'll see, you can be as profound or as abstract as you like! Be prepared to tailor how much you integrate the gift wrap into the body of your essay based on your topic. As a general suggestion, the more abstract subjects are best kept to the introductory and concluding fringes of your essay, while the more tangible the gift wrap, the easier it is to weave seamlessly throughout your essay. How thickly you layer it on is up to you; just make it consistent. You don't want to have more than one theme—the personal statement is too short and our goal is to give the essay one theme for the reader to remember it by.

Gift Wrap Example 1: Guinea Pig Tragedy
(more on the abstract side)

This student had recently experienced the death of a close friend's guinea pig. The experience made him think about how he approaches his medical education, so he chose this as his gift wrap.

Introduction:

Guinea pigs—unremarkable and mundane, or a role model for success?

On initial observation, guinea pigs don't tend to be highly regarded creatures; in fact, the cliché representation of the animals involves their use as initial trial subjects in exploratory scientific research. This common association with guinea pigs doesn't garner them much respect. So what do they have to do with physicians, or medicine?

Guinea pigs are animals that act based on their 'id,' acting within their abilities to obtain sufficient resources to survive according to their hierarchy of needs at the time. They are typically viewed as simple animals, but they still possess the same curiosity and drive to explore their environment that I think most medical students have. Guinea pigs also eat eclectic, but vegetarian diets—their favorite foods include alfalfa, hay, melon, oranges, spinach, and broccoli—which also represents an important quality in successful medical students: the ability to maintain an eclectic array of talents, interests, and perspectives while still adhering to a prescribed career path. Lastly, guinea pigs have been frequently known to persevere and maintain their typical upbeat and exploratory mood even in the most adverse circumstances. A personally poignant example involved a close friend's guinea pig, Squeakers...

Conclusion:

...Squeakers's situation reignited my thoughts on medicine; though guinea pigs may seem simple and unremarkable, they have some important qualities that I feel represent important attributes medical students and physicians should embody. Though medicine sometimes involves pain, death, and adversity, it is carries an intense, intrinsic reward that is unmatched by anything else I could pursue. Through Squeakers' bad fortune emerged a discovery that sometimes the seemingly unremarkable can be interesting and educational as well.

Gift Wrap Example 2: Social Interaction in Elevators
(midway between profound and abstract)

This student was very focused on international public health and felt that public health was the practice of medicine in distinct contexts. She uses her gift wrap to draw the reader in and begin her discussion of the importance of context, and thus of how she plans to practice medicine in international public health.

Introduction:

Why don't we speak to each other in elevators?

Throughout the innumerable elevator trips I have taken, one standard holds: the passengers, including myself, almost uniformly choose to watch the numbers light up instead of engaging in discourse. Perhaps we are avoiding meaningless interactions (so that we do not feel as meaningless?). Is there any point to asking how you are if I have no context in which to interpret your answer? Can I truly care about your answer without that context? If your answer is not 'fine,' will I be able to suggest anything without context? Intuitively, the answer to these queries is 'no' and points to why we would rather discuss the weather. Thus, even in our most insignificant interactions, context is far from insignificant.

Public health, in my eyes, embodies perhaps the most oft-asked question in the world, "How are you?" It is an inquiry into not only physical health, but also one's subjective state of being— really anything and everything that may affect someone. We perform this assessment on every level, from individual to global. Is any other field more inclusive in its examination of the human experience?...

Conclusion:

...Concordant with my personal background, these goals are international in scope. Globalization has limited our degrees of separation; the world is now a common elevator. How long does one take the elevator with the same people before the interaction becomes meaningful? I believe that my aforementioned perspectives are needed most in developing countries, and that developing environments are where such a shift in both clinical and public-health approaches would be most possible...

...By eventually applying these skills towards health and development, I hope, as a passenger on this elevator, to ensure our movement is upward.

4.2.5 Step 5: Outline!

This step is self-explanatory. Simply stated, the best essays are ones which flow naturally. Outlining before you write is key to good organization. Cheyenne's outline is below in **Figure 4.2.5a**, followed by her essay (**Figure 4.2.5b**).

Gift Wrap: Medicine is art analogy

I. **Introduction:** *medicine/art analogy*
   A. *Medicine is art*
   B. *Doctors are artists/restorers of art*

II. **Cardinal Question:** *Why me?*
   Motivation: *Neuroscience major*
   A. *I approach problems with an interdisciplinary/ comprehensive approach*
   B. *It taught me to work in teams*
   C. *It taught me to revere how amazingly unique each human is, which makes me appreciate the power of communication*
   D. *It reinforces how I have interacted with people from all walks of life/ travel/liberal arts school*

III. **Cardinal Question:** *Why medicine?*
   Experience: *Living in Italy/ Art*
   A. *Personal fulfillment from art and medicine—gives me same satisfaction/sense of achievement*
      1. *Painting in Lucca/ rendering Rosso's painting*
      2. *Counselling my schizophrenic patients/ figuring out hyaluronidase puzzle*
   B. *Both bring renewal—happy feeling and renewal of my desire and effort—more motivation*
   C. *Challenge—both make me adaptive and I will constantly be learning*
   D. *Betterment of humankind—both make us feel better*

III. **Conclusion:** *Want to be a doctor because it is the ultimate art form to me*

Figure 4.2.5a Sample Outline

I once overheard someone say, "Medicine is more regiment than art." This simple comment evoked an intricate chain of thoughts that had a powerful impact on me. Pondering such words has led me to clarify my personal outlook on the relationship between medicine and art, two very important influences in my life. As a premed student and an amateur artist, I have to strongly disagree with the above statement. I wholeheartedly believe that medicine is an art; it is the art of practicing health science. The human body is nature's greatest work of art, a notion held by renowned artists and scientists throughout history. Recognition of this concept inspired my interest in medical science. I marvel that not only in pure external form, but also in the amazing synchrony of mind and body, complex coordination of mental processes, and internal harmony, every human is a living masterpiece.

By this analogy, every doctor is an artist, perhaps even a restorer of art. I believe that just as art requires careful planning, innovation, self and peer critique, and subject evaluation, so with every diagnosis does medicine. As much as art demands hard work, time, commitment, and study, so too does medicine require passion, along with knowledge and discipline. With all the anomalies and exceptions to health, with new concerns and constantly mutating viruses, with the sheer concept of human uniqueness, medicine is not, and never will be, a practice of regiment. No human or great work of art is like another and, similarly, no two doctors or artists perform exactly alike; each will have his or her own stylized stroke of brush or scalpel.

Medicine, in the same vein as art, develops highly individualized skill while simultaneously upholding communal standards and traditional methodology. The interdisciplinary nature of my neuroscience major has instilled in me the value of teamwork and of confronting problems with a comprehensive approach. At the heart of my neuroscience studies lies the fact that the intimate feedback between the brain and environment makes it essentially impossible to separate the brain from the influence of the world that nurtures it. This truth ensures that we are not only unique physically, but also in our mental processes and conscious awareness. From this perspective, the ability to relate to another human being, to understand one another, becomes an ineffably breathtaking phenomenon. My reverence for this miraculous concept is further nourished by my liberal arts education, which fosters interaction in the same manner that my aesthetic studies further enable me to appreciate the human body. Medicine is the culmination of such links between art and science.

In drawing out my thoughts thus far, I realize that the strongest connection I can make between medicine and art is not theoretical but personal. After an entire semester in Italy immersed in art, I can now acknowledge that painting the landscapes of Lucca inspired within me the same profound exuberance as counselling my patients diagnosed with schizophrenia. Similarly, rendering Rosso Fiorentine's *Punto Musicale* and trying to elucidate the nature of hyaluronidase byproducts in mesolpothemia at Mt. Sinai Medical Center filled me with the same energy of purpose, the same excitement of achievement. The processes of performing art and the elements of medicine to which I have been exposed fulfill me inexplicably. The ultimate expression of this personal rapture and enchantment is renewal. Art and medicine renew my spirit through a sense of accomplishment and the everlasting opportunity to continue to learn and grow. Both art and medicine challenge me to be dynamic and adaptive to new techniques and obstacles, and both serve the betterment of humankind. The plausibility of healing others while renewing myself is fascinating. The direct purpose of helping one another is what makes medicine the ultimate form of art, the ultimate bridge between the humanities and the sciences, and thus the ultimate area of study. This is why I want to become an artist of the sciences, a doctor.

Figure 4.2.5b Sample Personal Statement
Note: The text in green corresponds to the green text in Cheyenne's Self-Reflection Chart (**Figure 4.2.3b**) above.

4.3 THE WRITING PROCESS—ANTICIPATING ROADBLOCKS

4.3.1 Paragraph Structure

It may have been a while since you last wrote an essay, so let's review paragraph basics. This is one of those things that won't win you points if you nail it, but will most certainly derail your admissions efforts if you ignore it.

- **One major idea per paragraph as a general rule**. Make sure you have a thesis statement to give the reader an idea of the subject matter. If you are on the fence about dividing a big paragraph into smaller ones, remember that shorter paragraphs are easier to digest and less intimidating on first glance.

- **Make sure you have smooth transitions from paragraph to paragraph.** There should be a flow to the essay, which comes from the organization you decided while designing your outline. A paragraph break is insufficient to herald the introduction of a new idea—part of your job is to hand-hold the reader through your message, which is harder if your structure is choppy.

4.3.2   Length

AMCAS only gives you 5,300 characters to write your personal statement: they say this is approximately one full page. Many of the examples you'll see here are slightly below or above that mark—obviously, constraints of the online application will force you to err on the shorter side—but at least you'll know that if you're still plugging away around the 4,900-character mark, you should start concluding your thoughts. Remember that sometimes less is more (refer to that section for details).

When describing your experiences, keep the exposition brief; it will help control your length. Cramming in an introduction of detailed biographical information every time you mention an experience will seem like a deluge of information to the reader. You should include only the details necessary to justify the relevance of the information. For example, if you're dying to talk about how shadowing an attending at Columbia Presbyterian had a profound impact on your career direction, you don't need to include which shifts you worked or your start/end dates. We realize that many of you may be hesitant to give the appearance of informlity by omitting details. Be assured that admissions readers are intimately familiar with routine procedures and assignments common to premed clinical experiences. Rote recitation of tedious details will distract your reader and make him or her less interested, or even worse, put off. You'll have your most important experiences listed in the extracurricular section of the AMCAS (or similar) application, so be reassured that if the reader insists on knowing the date you started your first volunteer shift, for example, he or she can look there for that information.

4.3.3 Quotes

Students like to have their thoughts supported by a quote from someone credible—usually someone famous. Quotes can be a valuable device to say something profound without sounding pretentious, or to make a statement without having to justify it. Quotes can help readers to put your thoughts into context, demonstrate that you can take a meaningful lead from a respected public figure, or that you have a sense of humor.

- **Don't use a quote just because you think you have to**. If you have a quote in mind before you start writing, that's great. However, quotes that are thrown in afterward or that have been worked in tangentially always stand out. Only use a quote if it truly helps you to get a point across.

- **Don't use famous quotes from famous public figures.** You're not going to be the first person to quote Gandhi, Martin Luther King, or William Osler. Quotes can be a useful addition to a statement, but unless you have a unique or quirky take on an oft-used quote, better to steer clear of those. Theese famous statements may have added a lot to society, but they're not going to fast track you into medical school.

Example of using a quote properly:

> Oddly enough, it was one of my favourite television actresses, Eva Longoria, who inspired me to reevaluate my life goals. Her words, "Passion is not something that can be bought or learned—it comes from the soul," made me realize what a gift it is, in a sometimes bleak world of obligation and dependence, to be able to experience passion for something. Pondering this led me to realign my career aspirations with my passions.

In this funnel introduction, the applicant uses the quote to lead into a series of ideas that make sense and are on a similar scale. Matching the scale of the quote with what you use it to talk about is important in making the quote seem like it belongs in your essay. For example, you wouldn't want to use a philosophical quote (grand scale) to talk about tying your shoes (small scale)—unless you were *trying* to be funny.

Example of poor quote usage:

> "An eye for eye only ends up making the whole world blind." Gandhi's insightful words on dealing with adversity were pivotal in moderating my interactions with difficult patients while volunteering in Miami Children Hospital's ER.

In the first example, the quote is an appropriate introduction to a meaningful thought. Although quoting a *Desperate Housewives* series regular in an intellectual context is risky, it connects to the applicant's situation in a way that is evocative and persuasive. If you can pull off making Eva Longoria sound profound and academic, using her over an over-quoted pundit will win you respect for taking a risk and succeeding.

The sentiment of the second quote is inappropriate for a personal statement; though this applicant likely had good intentions in quoting Gandhi, the quote, gives the impression that the applicant wants to retaliate against the patients but does not. This description of restraint will quickly send this applicant back to application-sending 101 (or even to a blacklist). A more appropriate description of dealing with difficult patients might portray the experience as unexpected and address engaging the patients in a positive manner (insight and growth *do* win big points!).

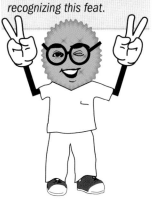

Refraining from harming patients is always a valiant choice, but medical schools don't yet have awards *recognizing this feat.*

4.3.4   Imagery

Imagery enriches the experience of sharing your thoughts with the reader and demonstrates your capacity for abstract thought and creativity. Strong images can help you to bring the reader to experience what you have. However, if you tend to overdo it (or don't know if you do), following these ground rules will help your essay to be profound and well-researched rather than over-the-top.

Root your imagery in something meaningful. It's a lot more meaningful to relate your feelings to something concrete (such as a concept, film, or book) and to give details of this relationship, rather than to use simple or groundless metaphors or other devices. Notice in the following examples how the first description reads much stronger than the second. In the first example, we feel like participants in this applicant's moment. In the second example, it's hard to empathize with the writer's decisions and passions because of the lack of context and believability in her imagery.

Example of good use of imagery:

> Every Thursday, I would spend the afternoon in the waiting room of my father's office. After the last patient left, my father would take me to his office, let me sit in his chair, and give me cookies. In Iran, a country where only a few can afford health care, my father would see most of his patients free of charge, and they would bring him pastries as a thank you gift. That was my first encounter with medicine: Sweet.

Example of overdone imagery:

> When I worked with my mom as a child at a geriatric facility, the seeds of passion for health care were implanted within me, and they continue to blossom in my veins; the feeling is indescribable. Making a career decision at the age of twelve required some rational explanations. Thus, I ventured into hospitals seeking answers.

The particular applicant quoted in the overdone example was trying to describe the impact of her exposure to patients in a geriatric nursing facility, where her mother was a nurse, on her decision to study medicine. The applicant later found a more personal, effective way to connect that exposure with a poignant memory of her grandmother:

> As my mother began the patient's I.V., she caressed the elderly lady's hand and said, "Her skin is so soft, so fragile." I recalled my grandmother, although with quite different sentiment. My own cheeks flushed as I revisited my younger self, rude and demanding, which brought tears down my grandmother's wrinkled cheeks.

4.3.5 The 'Fudge Factor'

"I can fudge?!..." Well, yes and no. We certainly do not advocate or condone fabricating details in a personal statement. However, we are aware that many of you, faced with the fear of being perceived as unsavory, might err on the modest side. In this process, fear can be an unwelcome, unexpected addition to the process that can alter your presentation of yourself on paper and in person. We've seen students err on the side of heavy modesty despite stellar achievements, and thankfully, fewer that erred on the bombastic side. Don't allow one cog in the wheel of medical school admissions (are you getting the imagery?) to derail years of effort that got you to where you are today. You've earned the right to apply to medical schools, so exercise it to the best of your ability. Let's draw some boundaries with an example.

Let's say you worked one summer at MGH (Massachusetts General Hospital), but you spent most of your days in a secluded laboratory doing HPLC runs for an attending that saw patients only on days when the barometric pressure was between 30-32 mmHg and winds were originating from the far northwest. Not a lot to wow medical schools with, right? Well, you did work at one of the world's top hospitals, so you've had significant

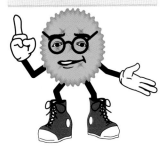

Don't make your decision to study medicine seem manipulated or contrived. Keep the sentiment; change the imagery!

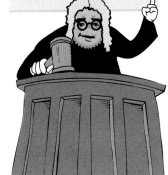

No notaries or sworn affidavits! Be relieved that MD/DO applicants don't have the reputation MBA applicants have—all top business schools require applicants to pay for application background checks!

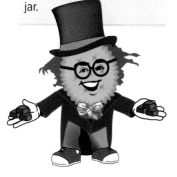

Embrace the Fudge Factor to let it work for you. Beware though: most applicants who fudge too much are caught with their hands in the cookie jar.

circumstantial exposure to clinical medicine. However, you didn't round with the plastic surgery team every morning. Based on this experience, it's okay to say that being surrounded by some of the world's top physicians, or seeing patients in varying states of health while walking around, had an impact on your perception of medicine (or motivations, etc.). You don't even have to mention or dwell on the monotonous HPLC runs. On the other hand, you cannot talk about the thrill of being in the operating room, doing procedures, etc. if you weren't there and didn't do it.

The devil is in the details, as they say. The variable you have to play with is the level of detail you provide.

4.3.6 Grammar Refresher

Now it's time to bring up a seemingly obvious point: use proper grammar. Well, duh. But "good grammar" is such a nebulous phrase that can be interpreted to mean almost anything. So, what about "good grammar" do you need to know to nail it for your personal statement?

Unfortunately, using good grammar is like having credit—it doesn't matter until it's used badly. You can skim this section if you're an English or writing major, or if you've won a Pulitzer. Otherwise, to avoid the bleak fate that befalls grammar-rule violators, keep these things in mind:

Every sentence should have a subject and verb. Just because we break this rule by using a bunch of sentence fragments and dangling antecedents doesn't mean you can. You're auditioning for a pedigree, so you need to appear refined enough to show potential to earn it. And part of creating that appearance means abiding by basic sentence structure. If you want to be more creative with your sentence structure, just be sure to run it by an English professor.

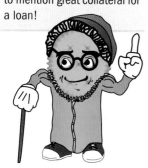

Yes, an MD is a pedigree... not to mention great collateral for a loan!

Keep a good ratio of 1 thought: 1 sentence. In other words, don't use run-on sentences. This isn't an exact science—if it were your creativity would be stifled—but separate your wonderful insights into active, separate sentences. Commas can separate two short sentences, but be parsimonious in using them for that purpose (see how that comma separated two subject/verb phrases?). Readers have a great capacity for attention, but it will start to wear thin if continually have to go back and figure out the point you were trying to make.

Example of a run-on sentence:

It was initially created at the geriatric facility and progressed as I sought positions like pre-med intern at New York Presbyterian Hospital, Florence Nightingale Nursing Home, Manhattan Rehab. & Wellness, Brigham & Women's Young Hospital, and etc., facilities where I tried to maximize my learning experience through immersing myself in all settings thoroughly so that I was able to closely observe the elderly and physicians alike, which allowed me to gain first-hand insight into the profession.

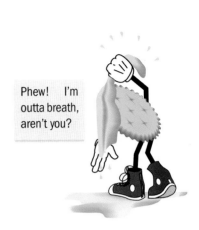

Phew! I'm outta breath, aren't you?

Now, folks, that's a run-on sentence. Obviously this poor writer didn't have the opportunity to read the 'less is more' section and insisted upon name-dropping an exhaustive work history into her statement. Even worse, it doesn't stop there—her stream of consciousness raced furiously towards joining downstream tributaries and became the mouth of the Mississippi (imagery, imagery!), drowning the reader's interest. Here's an improved version:

Example of good sentence-to-thought ratio:

It was initially created at the geriatric facility and progressed as I worked at various hospitals. At New York Presbyterian, I tried to maximize my learning experience through immersing myself in all settings thoroughly. Being able to closely observe the elderly and physicians alike allowed me to gain first-hand insight into the profession.

Avoid excess prose. Before you start your paragraph on how the lemon-scented cleaner on Founders 12 at HUP (Hospital of the University of Pennsylvania) awoke a fire in cranial nerve 1 that set motion to your olfactory centre and eventually inspired you to become a doctor, think about how to say this succinctly. Try starting a description using the bare minimum of details, evaluate its efficacy in conveying the message you want, and add any additional details necessary in a gradual fashion. For example, in the run-on sentence above, the applicant's insights were evident in the corrected statement even though many place names were removed. When you're ready, ask others: when someone else is able to extract your intended message from the sentence, then call it a day. Sometimes you will need include a lot of information, which is fine. But many times, you'll be able to trim the fat and demonstrate your organizational skills, too.

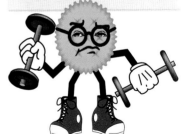

Savour the low-carb version of your thoughts.

Less is more. In addition to being wordy, people sometimes try to cram too much information into their personal statement. The whole reason we went through Step 3 (Connect-the-dots) is to select the information that is relevant and strategically plays into your message. So, really try to avoid including anything else. It's obvious when candidates are trying hard to squeeze in information. One especially annoying manifestation of this faux pas is what we affectionately term the "list technique."

Example of including irrelevant information:

> I also understood the importance of being a well-rounded person, attending a musical school and becoming a karate champion in one of the neighborhood championships, while maintaining excellent grades in school. The musical education, along with weekly piano lessons with my wonderful teacher, Mrs. Kaye, who taught students for 25 years, helped me to get in touch with my own emotions as well as to understand the feelings of others.

The above example demonstrates how personal statements can start to become a hodge-podge of unconnected information. Karate, music school, good grades, and a music teacher's qualifications are not placed into any meaningful context. Although the candidate is likely well-rounded and simply wants to express this fact, he ends up seeming arrogant and unfocused.

Don't give yourself away—if you practice karate or music only to be perceived as well-rounded instead of really enjoying these activities, don't tell the admissions committee!

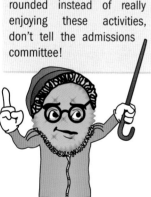

Example of "list technique":

> I play almost every sport there is: basketball, hockey, soccer, tennis, billiards, volleyball, swimming, snowboarding, rock-climbing, rafting, weightlifting, handball, racquetball, and occasionally baseball and football. As in my childhood, I try to keep up with new developments in the medical field by reading new articles during my spare time. I have also completed a semester of honors research in Professor Kramer's Lab, while being placed on the dean's list almost every semester and being inducted into the Golden Key Honour Society, which distinguishes the top 15% of undergraduate juniors and seniors worldwide.

We hope that by now you know exactly why this example is not the best use of the personal statement. This applicant uses valuable space to list activities he could have listed elsewhere, and he explains what is required to enter an honor society already well-known to medical schools. This applicant would have been better off talking about how sportsmanship related to his medical interests, or why his honors research was important to him. Instead, this applicant appears to be boastful, when, in reality, his achievements are common among other applicants to top medical schools.

4.3.7 Tone and Flow

Once you've completed the five steps and gone through the writing process, it's time to take a look at the tone and flow of your statement. Spell-checking and simply proofreading for grammar are not enough. Your essay should be a professional piece of work rather than a chit-chatty conversation. Let your personality shine through; however, nobody will feel comforted or impressed by slang statements (e.g. "I totally bugged out when my dad said he had a sixth digit.") Also, though you want to give the reader a window into 'you,' don't make your writing sound like an online dating profile.

Example of inappropriate tone:

> In my free time, I like to attend museums, Broadway shows, Devils games, various dance clubs, pursue my martial arts interest as much as possible and of course play sports. I also love to travel and explore new places. One of my lifelong dreams is to visit Europe with a bunch of my friends, which will hopefully come true this summer after I graduate.

Another grammar point that has a huge impact on tone is verb voice. Verb voice can be either active or passive. Look at the following sentences to see the difference, and guess which one is more effective:

- *"Having been present for the birth of my sister was something that changed my life."*

- *"As I watched the doctor deliver my baby sister, I immediately felt the sensation that this moment would change my life forever."*

The first sentence is written in passive voice, and the second one in active voice. The second statement is more vivid; the first is okay but isn't eye-catching. It's important to use more active descriptions and verbs in illustrating your experiences. It gives the impression that you are a more active, involved person who is more likely to take initiative in his or her education (*crucial* in medical education) rather than someone who waits around for life to happen.

When examining the tone of your essay, you should consider the flow in your assessment. We've already touched upon paragraph transitions, but it's also important to make sure ideas are introduced in a way that allows them to be addressed properly. New ideas introduced near the end of a statement don't allow for enough discussion of them—talk about them earlier, or not at all. Ensure that all your main ideas are introduced in the beginning of the essay, and that the body is used to flesh out your discussion not to rush through things. Many applicants change the organization of their original outline (Step 5) because they prefer the way the essay flows in a different order.

4.3.8   Proofreading

Who should proofread your essay and when? Different proofreaders will have different strengths in evaluating your statement, depending on their expertise. From our personal experience, we find it helpful to separate potential proofreaders into groups and to solicit individualized advice from each one.

Professors

Professors you know well are best (busy professors usually do this for their favorites), particularly if they are in the English department. Professors are great resources for determining the professionalism of your essay, as well as for focusing on grammatical points and structural issues. Their eyes are best attuned to critiquing those aspects of your essay; they may have other suggestions in terms of overall readability and general interest as well.

Friends

Though Rachel and Joey can't help you here, your non-TV friends, especially those not pursuing medicine or the sciences, are great for testing the readability of and general interest generated by your essay. Many admissions readers are career admissions officials, so the fact that they're working at a medical school has no correlation to their medical expertise or interest. People with a medical background may also read your personal statement, but their time is limited and the interest factor has an impact on their evaluation, too. Friends should tell you if your essay is incoherent or a snooze.

Writing/Career Services

Many universities have peer-run writing services or essay-consulting services through their career offices. Often, these services are also available to alumni of those institutions. This option is particularly helpful for those without the network to rely on professors; in most instances, the people chosen to run these services undergo a rigorous screening process so that their advice is meaningful and accurate.

You!

If you haven't reread your essay a few times, with some downtime in between (we've found overnight to be the minimum to let the material settle), then it's not ready. It's best to finalize your edits before you show your essay to friends and professors; you'll maximize your feedback potential from those sources by presenting them with a finished product, rather than relying on them for more substantial input on content and structure (something you should be doing yourself!).

Professional Services (Fee-Required)

There are quite a few professional essay-editing and writing services available. Our general advice is to avoid using these services unless you are truly unable to find a reliable third-party to take a look at your essay. Because these services have such varying reputations and levels of service (who knows if the client testimonial of the Harvard-accepted student is someone who just wanted an expensive spell-checker?), it's probably best to save your money. Thousands of students are admitted to medical schools without utilizing these services, so don't feel obligated to make this investment. However, if you have the financial resources, you could consider a full-service consultancy to walk you through the entire process (like utilizing the tools and tips in this book, but geared towards you personally) as an insurance policy. If you're going to pay for a third-party perspective, it will be more useful to you if the third party has as much background knowledge about you as possible.

4.4 GIVING YOURSELF ENOUGH TIME

How much time should you invest into this process? While the brainstorming and writing processes are very important, we know that everyone has different work habits. By the time you apply to medical school, you have probably already developed and discovered the work habits under which you produce your best work. However, there will always be people who turn everything upside down and change everything for this personal statement. Our advice—don't! If you always needed two weeks of steady progress to write a decent research paper, then take two weeks to compose your statement. If you have always benefited from the controlled panic of saving everything for the last minute, then don't change that. You want to be at your sharpest for this process—don't compromise your comfort zone if you can avoid it.

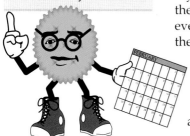

Just don't miss your deadlines!

If you haven't written an essay since you applied to undergrad, then you're probably a little rusty. Take some more time— even you procrastinators—to churn out a first draft. If you're the type of person who needs externally imposed deadlines, then get someone—your premed advisor, your classmate, your mom—to impose them. Even if the person reading it doesn't offer any constructive comments, by having written the draft you've gotten yourself back into composition mode and your second effort will be much better.

4.5 Non-traditional Applicants

If you have unusual or extenuating circumstances surrounding your application, including time off, working in other industries, poor science grades, etc., the personal statement is your opportunity to address these factors in a way not reflected in other parts of the application. You'll need to answer the cardinal questions in a different way than traditional applicants—you will need to create a flowing 'story' out of your experiences, particularly if your 'story' seems all over the place at first glance. Any negative circumstances, however, should be spun into positives if mentioned. For example, if you had poor grades freshman year, it's better to talk about this as a positive learning experience in time management and how you improved, rather than talking about having been overwhelmed by personal problems that semester. In general, medical schools love to see applicants come from unusual and interesting fields and circumstances; it's an easy way to add diversity to their ranks. However, the burden of addressing, and pitching, a less competitive record or explaining why you've switched to medicine rests solely upon you. Have fun with it! You're going to stand out, so do it in a positive way that will be remembered— maximize this opportunity by following the five steps.

Sample Non-Traditional Essay

This applicant's studies were interrupted multiple times by her father's debilitating illness. Reapplying to medical school, this applicant was faced with having to address her reasons for changing institutions and having gaps in her education and work history. She also had to persuade readers that these circumstances wouldn't cause any further interruptions (obviously, nobody can promise that a close family member won't die during medical school, but if her father is still sick and she plans on skipping every other week of class to be with him, readers will think it is too early for her to re-enter). She tied her reasons for switching schools to her personal tragedy—she argued that switching actually minimized interruptions and allow her to continue pursuing her dreams. Below is the result of her efforts, which shows how she followed the five steps and addressed the additional questions above. She chooses to discuss two experiences, her father's illness and attending medical school in the Caribbean, to answer the two cardinal questions.

Thankfully, many of you will not be faced with addressing such a weighty topic in your essay. Let the five steps guide your brainstorming, and remember to demonstrate insight and growth from anything negative you feel you must address.

Every Thursday I would spend the afternoon in the waiting room of my father's office. After the last patient left, my father would take me to his office, let me sit in his chair, and give me cookies. In Iran, a country where only a few can afford health care, my father would see most of his patients free of charge, and they would bring him pastries as a thank you gift. That was my first encounter with medicine: Sweet. Years later, while studying for my anatomy final at St. George's Medical School, I thought of those days.

My father received his residency training in New York. After his return to Iran, he founded the Republican Party of Iran, which advocated a free society like the one he had grown fond of, in the United States. After the revolution in Iran, my father, like many others who opposed the Khomeini regime, received death threats. He fled Iran and returned to the States. Since it was not safe to take a young child on such a trip, and my parents had divorced, my grandmother became my guardian. I did not see my father for the next ten years, since in Iran a girl under the age of eighteen is not allowed to leave the country without her father. A year after I graduated high school, my grandmother lost a long battle to cancer. A few months later, I arrived in New York, to see my father and continue my education. Then I found out about my father's illness. During my sophomore year in college, he underwent a brain surgery that left him hemiparalyzed.

In January of 2001 I left New York for Grenada to pursue a career in medicine. During the first session of my anatomy lab, I realized that I had found my calling. For the first time I was learning this profession's tools and language.

A few days before my finals, I received a call from New York regarding my father. He had suffered from a seizure and was

---

hospitalized. His condition had worsened, and he could not walk any longer. Since we had no other family members in the States, I decided to return. I discussed my situation with Prof. Rao, St. George's School of Medicine's Dean. He recommended that I leave as soon as possible and take my final exams upon my return to Grenada in August. Since my anatomy exam was only days away and the course had an extensive lab component, I was not able to take that exam before leaving for New York.

A few weeks after my return, my father was discharged from the hospital. I spent the rest of the summer caring for him, hoping that with therapy he would be able to walk again. By August it was clear to me that my father's condition had not improved to the point that he could care for himself. I contacted Dr. Rao, asking him for a year of leave of absence, so that I could help my father. Dr. Rao was supportive of my decision.

During the summer of 2002, with the help of social workers and my father's physicians, he finally qualified to receive homecare. Even though he could not walk any longer, he was able to care for himself with the help of an aid. I was to leave New York for Grenada on the 10th of August; I had been studying during the summer and was looking forward to resuming my medical education. In the early hours of July 22nd, my father woke me up, telling me that he felt he was about to die. After the emergency room visit, late the MRI revealed that his tumor had grown, taking over more than half of the frontal lobe. He was given less than two months to live. Soon after he was stripped of any ability to walk or speak.

Then I made an important decision to devote myself to making the most of the precious time I had left with my father. I undertook the role of his advocate and sole caregiver. As much as I loved my studies, I informed Dr. Rao that I would stay in New York to care for my father. I postponed my dreams, but never forgot my ultimate goal. I immersed myself in reading about my father's condition and worked closely with his doctors. My father is still with me; even his doctors are surprised. Even though most people cannot understand him when he speaks, I am one of the lucky few who can. He has told me many times just how much he wants to live and hopes to overcome his illness. During the last year, I have learned a lot about myself and the profession of my choice. My father's endurance and love of life has taught me how precious life is. The things that I have learned both as a patient's family member and as my father's only voice have, if anything, strengthened my determination to pursue a career in medicine. And after spending a semester in medical school, I feel that in a way, I have been on both sides now. These difficult times were also a time of self-examination for me, as I have learned a lot about myself and my abilities to overcome crisis.

While trying to find a treatment that might save my father's life, I have had the honor of meeting very accomplished physicians. Although I have respected physicians since my childhood, my experiences have left me with profound respect for this profession. They have taught me that in addition to the scientific aspects of medicine, it is important to understand a patient's and family members' frustrations, and their feelings of hope and fear. I have learned that medicine is about healing, not fixing. And a healer must be compassionate and empathetic in caring for patients.

I believe that my academic performance is evidence of my intellectual ability to undertake the learning of the scientific knowledge of medicine. In addition, my experiences have left me with dedication, humility, and a love of humanity, the elements that make medicine a human science.

My experiences, and much more importantly, what I have learned from them—I refer to them as "my life lessons in medicine"—have enabled me to bring a unique view of life and the art of healing to this noble profession. I have already taken the Hippocratic Oath, and feel fortunate to have found my purpose. For as Sir William Osler once said, "The practice of medicine is an art, not a trade; a calling, not a business; a calling in which your heart will be exercised equally with your head."

Figure 4.3 Sample Non-Traditional Essay

·

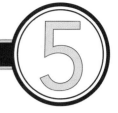

SECONDARY APPLICATIONS

5.1 HOW IMPORTANT ARE THEY?

Secondary applications should be far from 'secondary' on your list of priorities. Secondaries are your chance to let each particular school know why you are applying. You've already presented your argument as to why you're right for medical school when you answered the two cardinal questions, and now you must target your research and essays to each individual institution.

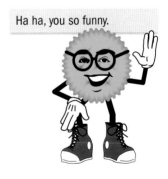

Ha ha, you so funny.

A typical secondary will include a few short-answer questions and a longer essay and will have a wider variety of questions than the primary. As a result, schools will tend to place greater value on the material submitted with the secondary, since it's less 'cookie-cutter' than the AMCAS application. Many institutions send secondaries to anybody who submits a primary application, so the competition remains intense in Phase 2. So don't lose steam here—the process is step-wise and predictable, and we'll guide you through it.

5.1.1 Examples of Some Secondary Questions

Longer Essays

> *Describe an ethical dilemma you encountered and how you handled it. What did you learn from this experience?*

Describe a challenge or obstacle you have faced and how you overcame it.

Short Answer

What extracurricular activity held the most significance for you and why?

What is your favourite book and why?

Secondary-application questions are not frequently changed; schools tend to have a signature question that they ask year after year. Because of this, most schools know what the others ask and try to make their questions unique. This means a whole lot of writing; few of your responses will be reusable for other applications. Use the information and lessons from **Chapter 4** to guide your writing.

5.2 How to Tackle Secondaries

5.2.1 Referring Back

Before you even start writing anything in the short- and long-answer boxes, revisit the materials you submitted with your primary application. You should review the qualities and events in your life that you highlighted throughout the primary application, mini-statements and all. These will be facets of 'you' that you should continue to expand upon in your secondary application. Go through the self-reflection chart you created and review your strengths and weaknesses. The answers to your secondaries will mostly come right off of your self-reflection chart. Another advantage of referring back is that your story and message will be consistent. You can imagine a red flag would be raised if an applicant gushed about public health in the primary application but professed his love for plastic surgery in the secondary. By all means, expose different facets of yourself, just don't contradict yourself.

5.2.2 Researching Schools II: Institution-targeted Responses

Many of the questions in your secondary application are there to ascertain the reason you have an interest in a particular institution. Of course, all aspects of the application help admissions gauge your personality and creativity as well. Use the strategies you used for the primary application—the two cardinal questions—as a guide to your approach. However, replace 'medical school' in the second cardinal question with 'Vanderbilt' or 'UCLA' or whichever school(s) interests you.

In order to do this without sounding generic or contrived, you will need to spend some time on the internet researching institutions. To be effective and specific, you should be scouring each school's website for curricula, departmental information, offerings, student opportunities, and past accomplishments. For example, if you are really interested in international health, when you're looking at a particular school, check to see if there are physicians doing international work (some schools actually have global-health departmental websites, where you can get information on how many students have had international experiences and where). You want your reasons for attending a particular school to have both breadth and depth and to show that you are making a mature and informed decision; some research is required to get your responses to that level.

A good way to target a school effectively and with less effort is to find out what a particular school thinks is unique about itself, and if you value that quality, highlight it. Many schools have qualities they think are differentiators, aspects of their institution on which they place a premium. For example, Yale prides itself on having a unique curriculum which gives students a competitive edge when applying to residencies. Even though anybody who spends more than thirty seconds on the Yale website can figure this out, it's still efficacious to use aspects a school prides itself on in order to target your secondary applications. For example, you could say, "Having the opportunity for more elective time, I'll be able to make a more informed decision on which specialty will best serve my interests in urban health." See how the applicant didn't just regurgitate that the curriculum was unique? Tailoring your pitch requires more thought than just cutting and pasting. Over time and through research, it will become progressively easier to identify differentiators for each institution in which you are interested and to determine if and how it fits with what you want out of your medical education.

Don't tell Harvard that you're applying there because it has a good reputation—everybody knows that. Be as specific and unique as you can.

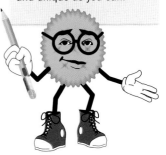

Individual School Websites
Partial Index: http://www.usnews.com/usnews/edu/grad/directory/dir-med/dirmedindex_brief.php

Table of Online Resources

5.2.3 Short & Sweet

Be concise in your responses. Many short-answer questions have word guidelines or limits; though you don't need to adhere to them strictly (unless it's in a text box online that counts characters inserted, nobody is going to sit and count), readers will be able to sense if your replies are long or if you are too verbose. In general, don't exceed word limits by more than 10-15 words. Being verbose might not only cause the reader to snooze, it will also lead them to question whether you have the ability to identify and highlight pertinent information when answering a question. Triaging and targeting information is 70% of what you will do as a medical student and as a physician, and you should show schools you know how to prioritize. It's okay to be below the word limit; readers will be grateful to you for having saved their time. In addition, they've probably "heard it all before" anyway.

5.2.4 Let Your Personality Shine Through

Have fun! Having fun in this process will loosen you up and give schools a better window into who you are than if you are anxious or hesitant in your responses. Students who appear to have genuine, focused interests (particularly those not normally pursued by premeds) are highly sought after by admissions committees. The primary application is the place to connect your eclectic personal experiences with medicine in general; the secondaries are where you need to connect the 'genuine, wonderful you' with a particular institution.

You don't want to talk about waking up in a supermarket parking lot after a crazy night of partying. But you can talk about your band's road trip—just keep it G-rated and relevant.

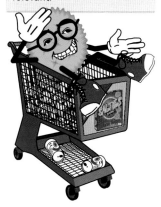

5.3 Maximizing the Efficacy of Secondaries

After all this, you're probably thinking, "How do I make this work?" Keep these tips in mind:

- Focus on one main interest or goal. Keep other interests more peripheral, as not doing so tends to complicate things (though by no means omit them, particularly if they show depth, breadth, and commitment, and especially if you don't know any other pre med who shares those interests).

- Find at least one differentiator (unique perceived strength) for each school.

- Target your short- and long-answer questions to the differentiator you've identified for each individual school.

- Refer back to your self reflection chart to refamiliarize yourself with your strengths, interests, and goals, particularly if it's been a while.

- Check and re-check your responses for clarity, diction, and verbosity

The secondaries are your chance to secure an interview—give them all you've got!

PREPPING FOR THE INTERVIEW

6.1 NAILING YOUR INTERVIEW

Okay, so this is the final cut! This phase of the admissions process is the most important deciding factor for *where* you end up going to medical school. The good news is that if you've been offered a few interviews, you are most likely going to be accepted somewhere; medical schools accept 25-50% of applicants they interview.

6.1.1 The Importance of Interview Performance

Interviewing is intense because it involves grooming everything about yourself. On at least a subconscious level, you are going to be judged by the interviewers. So you should strive to neutralize their subconscious judgment by conforming to a conservative version of yourself (or maybe you already are conservative). People wear blue or black suits, don dress shoes and pantyhose, and even remove piercings and cover tattoos for interview season. The medical preffesion is still very conservative, and there is no getting around that. There is a certain old-school conception about what a doctor should be like, and in any culture, a doctor is expected to be an upstanding member of society. The medical institution seeks to uphold that image. Paradoxically, you are simultaneously supposed to make yourself stand out from other

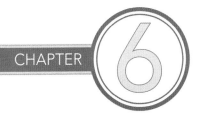
No miniskirts or mohawks!

applicants and show yourself to be an out-of-the-box-thinker! The inherent contradiction in trying to be unique while trying to fit in makes interviewing tough. To sail through these varying demands of interviews, you need to have a solid sales pitch.

6.1.2   What's a Sales Pitch?

Simply stated, your sales pitch is your story. Not your story of getting stuck in traffic on the way to the interview or spilling mocha latte on your blouse, but the story of what drew you to medicine and why you should be practicing it. A sales pitch is your story strategically emphasized and glamorized to demonstrate that you are an ideal candidate. (Most successful candidates have a sales pitch without even realizing it.) Your goal is to develop your story into a nicely rounded presentation of your qualities and ambitions in medicine, and then tighten it up and practice it until you know it backwards and forwards like a sales pitch.

6.2 The 'Six Platinum Steps' to a Savvy Sales Pitch

The good news is that all the work you put into developing your personal statement in **Chapter 4** is going to payoff when you develop your sales pitch. If you didn't use this book to write your personal statement, please go through the exercises in Steps 1 & 2 in **Chapter 4** (Section 4.2.1–4.2.2). It really won't take much time and it will provide a useful foundation for your sales pitch. Your pitch will be well coordinated with your personal statement, but it goes a step beyond. We're going to walk you through this process, continuing with our representative student, Ms. Cheyenne Ng Starr, from **Chapter 4**.

6.2.1   Step 1: Review Your Brainstorm for the Cardinal Questions

Remember the two cardinal questions (**Chapter 4**, Section 4.2.1): Why do you want to be in medicine? Why does medicine want you? Please review your brainstorms to these questions. Even though it's only been a few months since you brainstormed your answers, you may want to quickly check in with yourself to make sure your answers still match how you feel at this point in the process. Below is Cheyenne's brainstorm, which we presented earlier in **Chapter 4**:

Why Medicine?	*Why Me?*
• *Healing is important to me* • *Ayurvedic-healing family background* • *Human body is the ultimate form of art to me*	• *Creative* • *Passionate* • *Approach medicine as an art* • *Approach problems from many different angles— interdisciplinary* • *Care about betterment of humankind*

Figure 6.2.1a: Cheyenne's Brainstorm to the
First 2 Cardinal Questions

6.2.2 Step 2: The Third Cardinal Question: *What Do You Want to Accomplish in Medicine?*

Okay, don't get scared! You don't have to know exactly what you want to do for the next four years. This is just theoretical, so dream a bit. If you could do anything, and you didn't have to worry about any external factors, what type of medicine would you go into? Why? In an ideal setting, what would you want to accomplish in that field? Would you open a free clinic in a rural area? Become an international flying surgeon with Operation Smile? Join Doctors Without Borders? Open a small private practice? Do research in proteonomics? Think big. Now, out of all your grand ideas, pick one. Select the one you are most interested in now. Don't worry; you're not committed for life. In fact, most students do not go into the specialty they envisioned when applying. However, your sales pitch needs a clearly defined goal to complete the story. So, without any stress, brainstorm the details of your selected goal by asking yourself who/what/where/how?

Medical schools are seeking goal-oriented and ambitious candidates. Having one consistent goal as part of your story demonstrates your focus and ability to plan ahead. It's a widely recognized fact that people with clearly defined goals are more likely to succeed. By being able to demonstrate a clearly laid out path of ambition, you too will be seen by your interviewer as more likely to succeed.

You may have already brainstormed this in your self-reflection chart (**Chapter 4**, Section 4.2.2).

Ms. Starr's Self-Reflection Chart is presented again below (**Figure 6.2.6b**), as she draws from this heavily to develop her sales pitch. She took a look at her "Goals in Medicine" brainstorm in her chart before answering the third cardinal question (highlighted in blue in the chart below). She was able to look at this list in the context of the first two cardinal questions, and this helped her narrow down her selection to infectious diseases and public health. She chose these two as her ambition because they made the most sense with her answers to the first two cardinal questions, and because they were the ones she truly felt the most interested in. Infectious disease is a specialty heavily tied to public health, so she was able to tie these two together as one goal. Cheyenne then had to use her imagination and consider the questions above. When she thought about what in infectious diseases/public health she would like to achieve, she immediately thought about working in HIV/AIDS. HIV/AIDS is a popular health topic these days, and a broad one; she had to find something more specific about HIV/AIDS that drew her to it. Below is her brainstorm on the third cardinal question:

Ambitions in Medicine: infectious diseases/public health

More specifically: HIV/AIDS

Even more specifically, who/what/where/how?

- involved in clinical care, as well as policy change and program development

- internationally, Africa or Asia because need is greatest there and I want to continue working in an international context

- focus on emphasizing the importance of nutrition and stress management in immune function for HIV-positive patients....maybe work to develop a more comprehensive care program that includes more holistic approaches, which can be delivered in a low-resource setting

- do this maybe by working in US govt framework (e.g. CDC, PEPFAR) or by starting my own NGO

Figure 6.2.2 Sample Brainstorm to the
Third Cardinal Question

6.2.3 Step 3: Put the Answers to the Three Cardinal Questions in Story Form

Tie your answers to the first two cardinal questions to your chosen medical ambition. Your answers to the first two cardinal questions form the part of the story that tells the interviewer *how you got here*. The answer to the third cardinal questions tells the interviewer where you are going to go *from here*. How do your reasons for going to medical school relate to your goals in medicine? Consider this with an emphasis on inward reflection and personal growth.

For Cheyenne, this was simple because she had chosen her goal in medicine with her answers to the first two cardinal questions in mind. Below you can see how her answers to the first two cardinal questions feed right into her chosen ambition (answer to third cardinal question) to form a story that is believable (and thus marketable!). Cheyenne selected parts of her answers to the first two cardinal questions that related to her chosen ambition (highlighted in pink text). Next, she elaborated on her third cardinal question brainstorm (in blue text below). Lastly, she took all this information and put it into the form of a story, while balancing being specific and being succinct. We left her sales pitch in bullet format so you can really see how she strings together her ideas smoothly, in an order that makes sense. It may be a good idea for you to do this as well—keeping your sales pitch in these bite-size pieces will facilitate weaving it into your responses. Each thought is numbered, so that you can see how they were reorganized in the alternate storyline below (**Figure 6.2.3b**).

First Cardinal Question: *Why medicine?*

- Healing is important to me
- Ayurvedic/holistic-healing family background
- Human body is the ultimate form of art to me

Second Cardinal Question: *Why me?*

- Creative
- Passionate
- Approach medicine as an art
- Approach problems from many different angles—interdisciplinary
- Care about betterment of humankind

Third Cardinal Question: *What do I want to accomplish?*

- infectious diseases/ public health—intimately connected fields, as ID plays into public-health programs and policies
- HIV/AIDS—one of the most aggressive infectious diseases of our time; plays into complex social dynamics and sensitive topics

---

- involved in clinical care, as well as policy change and program development—I view policy and programmatic development as the foundation for sustainable change.
- internationally, Africa or Asia—because need is greatest there and I want to continue working in an international context
- focus on emphasizing the importance of nutrition and stress management in immune function for HIV positive patients….maybe work to develop a more comprehensive care program that includes more holistic approaches and can be delivered in a low-resource setting

Cheyenne's Sales Pitch:

1. I'm interested in pursuing a career in infectious diseases and public health because I am drawn to the challenge in these two fields to learn and adapt constantly, to be a creative problem-solver, and to incorporate interdisciplinary approaches.

2. Since infectious diseases top health concerns in developing settings, the field is intimately connected with public health programs and policies. Through public health, I am able to uphold the Ayurvedic principles of holistic healing and sustainability that I was raised with.

3. I'm looking forward to being involved in policy change and program development in addition to clinical care —I view policy and programmatic development as the foundation for sustainable change.

4. More specifically, I would like to work in HIV/AIDS, one of the most aggressive infectious diseases of our time; plays into complex social dynamics and sensitive topics

5. I see myself working internationally in Africa or Asia—both because need is greatest there and I want to continue working in an international development context.

6. It's sad to me that current treatment of HIV-positive patients does not focus on holistic care, including stress management and nutrition.

7. I would like to focus on incorporating the importance of nutrition and stress management in maximizing immune function for HIV-positive patients. I'd like to

> not only develop a more comprehensive care program that includes such holistic approaches, but also one that may be effectively delivered in a low-resource setting.
>
> 8. Holistic approaches are especially important to take advantage of in low-resource settings, where ARVs may be unavailable.
>
> 9. Conquering HIV will take more than ARVs; we have to address stigma and access issues to have more effective prevention. Furthermore, prevention and treatment need to be culturally appropriate. I look forward to moving the global response to HIV/AIDS towards these goals.

Figure 6.2.3a Sample Story Developed from Answers
to the Three Cardinal Questions

Now, just for fun, we reorganized Cheyenne's thoughts to form an alternate storyline. We do this to demonstrate that the order of the information doesn't matter. All that matters is that you get the information across in a coherent fashion. The truth is you will be separating and reordering these thoughts as you mold them into your responses to interview questions. You may want to practice doing this yourself, to better hone your ability to lead into your sales pitch from any angle.

The two little changes Cheyenne made in reordering her thoughts are in red text.

> 6. It's sad to me that current treatment of HIV-positive patients does not focus on holistic care, including stress management and nutrition.
>
> 7. I would like to focus on incorporating the importance of nutrition and stress management in maximizing immune function for HIV positive patients. I'd like to not only develop a more comprehensive care program that includes such holistic approaches, but also one that may be effectively delivered in a low-resource setting.
>
> 5. I see myself working internationally in Africa or Asia—both because need is greatest there and I want to continue working in an international development context.
>
> 2. Since infectious diseases top health concerns in developing settings, the field is intimately connected

with public-health programs and policies. Through public health, I am able to uphold the Ayurvedic principles of holistic healing and sustainability that I was raised with.

3. I'm looking forward to being involved in policy change and program development in addition to clinical care—I view policy and programmatic development as the foundation for sustainable change.

8. Holistic approaches are especially important to take advantage of in low-resource settings, where ARVs may be unavailable.

1. In short, I'm interested in pursuing a career in infectious diseases and public health because I am drawn to the challenge in these two fields to constantly learn and adapt, to be a creative problem-solver, and to incorporate interdisciplinary approaches.

4. More specifically, I would like to work in HIV/AIDS, one of the most aggressive infectious diseases of our time; plays into complex social dynamics and sensitive topics

9. Conquering HIV will take more than ARVs; we have to address stigma and access issues to have more effective prevention. Furthermore, prevention and treatment need to be culturally appropriate. I look forward to moving the global response to HIV/AIDS towards these goals.

Figure 6.2.3b Alternate Storyline

6.2.4 Step 4: Add 'Flava'!

Bookmark which of you *experiences* and *qualities* play a role in this story and weave them in. The most important part of this exercise is to know *where* and *how* your experiences and qualities play into your story. Often these correspond to your answers to secondaries, and interviewers may ask you to go into more detail, so be ready to talk about them.

Cheyenne simply highlighted all the stuff in her self-reflection chart that was relevant to her story (highlighted in blue in **Figure 6.2.4** below). If there is a way something in your self-reflection chart can feed into your story, include it! This will give you more angles from which to enter your sales pitch. Below, we show how Cheyenne started to think of incorporating her self-reflection chart into her story.

Personal characteristics:

- Multidisciplinary approach to problems → incorporate immunology, nutrition, antiviral approaches to combating HIV
- Leadership → designing programs and policy
- Always growing & learning → need to constantly incorporate research into clinical practice; medicine is an ever-evolving field
- Care about betterment of humankind → healing people, more than just masking their symptoms; work at the level of communities and incorporate prevention education
- Creative → problem solver; look for innovative ways to approach the problem
- Many languages → international career; realize the great effect of culture on perception of health and disease

Experiences:

- Prefer working with patients/human interaction → why I want to have a clinical practice-community clinic for people living with HIV
- International travel → international career; already comfortable living and working abroad

Anything else:

- Grandma was an Ayurvedic healer and midwife → I grew up with the concept of holistic healing; this approach to health care is second nature to me
- Healing is a holistic process—must consider the whole person, not just the ailment → this is why antiretroviral therapy alone is not enough. Important to address all the other factors affecting the target organ and the immune system, such as nutrition, mental health, environment, etc.

Stuff not in the chart that I just thought of:

- Interesting articles I read for class on effects of stress and nutrition on immune function—stress and nutrition must be important factor for immune-compromised patients.

Figure 6.2.4 Sample of Weaving Additional
Self-Reflection Chart Contents into Story

6.2.5   Step 5: Be Able to Tell the Whole Story in 5 Minutes or 50

This isn't as tricky as it sounds. It's very possible to tell your story (answers to the three cardinal questions strung together in story form) in five minutes. But look at all the aspects of your personality and experiences that you can go into from the step above! If you touched on each of these topics, you could theoretically speak for a long time and still be telling one cohesive story.

Why do you need to prepare for a range of speaking time? Well, because each interview is unique (although they may start to seem the same after a while!). Interviews can have many different structures. You may not have much 'airtime' in a group interview; however, another interview could be a one-on-one conversation for an hour an a half! By clearly identifying the core of your sales pitch, and the add-ins, you can condense or extend your sales pitch accordingly.

Another way to extend your speaking time is to expand on your ambition. Since your ambition is just a dream, you can get as carried away with it as you like. Below are some ideas on ways in which to elaborate your ambition. Under each example, in blue text, are Cheyenne's brainstorms on how she would link her ambition to the following topics:

- Research you would like to engage in while in medical school
  I may want to do qualitative research on nutrition and stress in HIV-positive patients, linking this data to their CD4 counts or other physiological markers. I can refer to some studies I read in a biology class on the effects of stress and nutrition on immune function.

- Related rotations you will gear toward your goal
  rotations in public health, infectious diseases, HIV/AIDS; maybe an MPH joint program

- Organizations you would like to belong to, or start
  international health group, community HIV/AIDS-awareness group

- How your ambition ties into your personal growth
  Through this ambition, I can further my interest and motivations in holistic health care, travel, about learning other cultures, and sustainable change. At the same time, I get to make a unique contribution to addressing a population in need; this will no doubt be fulfilling.

6.2.6 Customize Your Pitch for Each School (Researching Schools III)

Figure out what aspects of a school will be important for your goal. For example, if you want to be a cardiothoracic surgeon, you should look for information such as the strengths of the school's surgery department, the percentage of students going into surgery residencies, etc. This is the information you should try to research *before* your interview. From your research, pick out characteristics of the school that *support* your ambition. You may stumble upon aspects of a school that do not support your ambitions; use this information when you are choosing between schools, but don't bring it up in an interview. You don't want to put down a school during your interview. Highlighting facets of the school that support your ambitions in medicine will show that you have a serious interest in the school and further your reputation as someone with a plan. Any information that you cannot find can be turned into a question for your interviewer (ahh, it's all coming together now). By turning a lack of knowledge into a relevant question about the school, you can obtain information which will help you to choose between schools *and* help you to appear goal-oriented and interested in that specific institution.

This research does not have to be extensive. We recommend doing this the day before your interview so that the information is fresh in your mind. After all, many people do stick to their plan when they enter medical school. The more serious you are about your chosen ambition, the more helpful this information will be in deciding which school to attend. It's also a good time to review general strengths and weaknesses of the school, the curriculum, and average student debt, just to have these aspects in mind in case you get the chance to ask questions of current students. If you do make inquiries of current students, seek answers that will help you choose between schools. Don't forget, you are also supposed to be evaluating the school during this trip, not just the other way around.

Below, we can see how Cheyenne customized her pitch for Cornell University Medical College.

Now she can tie in this research on the school whenever a relevant topic comes up during the interview. (It is common for topics in your personal statement to be a nidus of conversation during an interview.) For example, if her study abroad in Italy comes up, Cheyenne can lead into how she would like to work abroad. She may then mention her unsuccessful attempt at researching the availability of international clinical rotations and ask the interviewer for this information. Alternatively, she could have led into how she next wishes to live in India because it is a second-wave country in the HIV epidemic. From here she could go into her ambitions in the field of HIV and how great CUMC's HIV Clinic is. Since you have this strategic information (related to your ambition) on the school fresh in mind, you can easily weave this research into your conversation.

Cheyenne brainstormed the following relevant aspects of a school, which she researched online the night before interviewing:

- joint MPH program (she had looked into this in Phase 1, too)
- international rotations possible
- infectious disease rotations
- HIV/AIDS-related program

Here is what she found out about CUMC:

- joint MPH program

  1 yr MPH possible at Columbia between 3rd and 4th years

- international rotations possible
  She didn't find any information on this.

- infectious disease rotations
  Not only could she do an ID rotation, but they also offer a pediatric ID rotation.

- HIV/AIDS-related program
  CUMC's hospital has an entire HIV clinic that specializes in the latest clinical approaches to HIV care and pediatric HIV cases.

Figure 6.2.6a Sample Sales-Pitch Customization

	COLUMN 1: EXPERIENCES	COLUMN 2: PERSONAL CHARACTERISTICS	COLUMN 3: MOTIVATION
	Clinical	**Strengths**	**Goals in Medicine**
Basic Information	• Landmark Medical Center; Counselling Intern; Inpatient facility for schizophrenic inpatients; fall 1998 • Amgen; Genetic counselling intern; counselled high-risk pregnancies; spring 1998 • St. Josephs Medical Center; volunteer; helped with pediatric patients; spring 1996	• Multidisciplinary approach to problems • Teamwork/Communication • Leadership • Funny • Spiritual • Always growing & learning • Care about betterment of humankind • Passionate • Creative	• Neurology • Psychiatry • Infectious diseases • Public Health • Not sure • Not Research!
Lessons Learned	• Like counselling • Realized patients make decisions based on different value systems than docs		
	Extracurricular Experiences	**Weaknesses**	**Inspirational Figures**
Basic Information	• **Living in Italy** • **Art/Painting** • Spoken word/poetry • Dancing • International travel: India, Europe, South America • Collegians for Youth • South Asian Students Association	• Family! Lots of personal obstacles • Cultural obstacles being a first-generation woman • Lack of patience • Stubborn/lack flexibility • Don't like authority • Get bored fast	• Grandma— Ayurvedic healer and midwife

Lessons Learned	• *Art and medicine make me feel the same sense of fulfillment* • *Medicine is just like art to me*	• *Drawing boundaries* • *Seeking positive company (including other powerful women)* • *Communication*	• *Healing is a holistic process—must consider the whole person, not just the ailment* • *Natural approaches to healing*
	Research	**Quirks**	**Other Interests**
Basic Information	• *Mt. Sinai Medical Center; Volunteer Lab Assistant; studying Hyaluronidase cancer markers; summer 2000*	• *Many languages* • *Great bartender*	• ***Neuroscience major*** • *Viral oncogenesis* • *HIV/AIDS*
Lessons Learned	• *Don't like lab setting! Prefer working with patients/ human interaction*	• *Appreciate different cultures* • *Appreciate a good drink!* • *Learned that people always want someone to talk to*	• *May relate to my specialty in future?* • ***Amazed at how unique we are in brain function/ personality...works of art!*** • *Amazed by the power of both nature and nurture on personal development*

Figure 6.2.6b Cheyenne's Self-Reflection Chart
(with sales pitch relevant context highlighted)

http://services.aamc.org/currdir/section2/start.cfm (curricula) http://www.aamc.org/md2 (financial aid advice)

Figure 6.2.6c Table of Online Resources

6.3 DELIVERING THE PITCH

Okay, so you don't want to walk in and take over the room with your sales pitch. There is a fine line between proactive and pushy. You need to spend the first few minutes of the interview feeling out the interviewer's style. They expect to be directing the interview; however, many are open to applicants participating in shaping the interview. If an interviewer has a set of questions for you, then you will have to just incorporate your sales pitch, piece by piece, into your answers. On the other hand, the interviewer may actually offer you time to give your pitch (e.g. "Why don't you tell me a little bit about yourself and why you are applying to medical school?") You'll have to play it by ear. The key to doing this successfully is being so comfortable with your sales pitch that you can lead into it from many different angles. You may present more information than was originally in your pitch, depending on the questions you are asked. However, the answers to the questions medical schools are really interested in will come from your sales pitch. So get comfortable presenting your entire sales pitch, as well as presenting it piecemeal. It is likely that you will end up using both approaches during your interviews.

Below, we provide examples of leading into a sales pitch using our representative student, Cheyenne. The commentary after each question-answer example contains several important pointers for delivering your sales pitch. We've used a few common interview questions, so you can practice leading into your sales pitch with these questions, too!

An important skill is being able to see how a question relates to your sales pitch. In the examples below, we 'translate' the questions (*in italics*) to reveal which aspects of a sales pitch the question is targeted toward. The whole reason we discuss the three cardinal questions is because the majority of interview questions relate to them. This should come as no surprise as the whole purpose of an interview is to investigate your answers to the three cardinal questions. Understanding this concept is key to being able to successfully prepare for interviewing. Practice identifying which cardinal question the examples below relate to. Even seemingly unrelated questions can be pretty easily linked to one of the cardinal questions. For example, a question intended to challenge you (e.g. Please explain nuclear fission) is really allowing the interviewer to assess how you function under stress, as this is an important part of being a doctor. This type of question is related to the second cardinal question: *Why should medical schools want me?*

Example 1: Question related to why you chose to go into medicine and your influential figures

> **INTERVIEWER:**
> Were you influenced by relatives to pursue a career in medicine?
>
> **CHEYENNE:**
> Actually, yes! My grandmother is an Ayurvedic healer, so I was raised with the concept of holistic healing. Approaching health holistically is a great part of my ambition in medicine.

This questioner may have really intended to weed out candidates who are just going into medicine because mommy and daddy are docs and told them to become the same. However, Cheyenne took the opportunity to bring up two aspects of herself (influenced by grandma and into holistic healing) from her sales pitch. More importantly, she dropped the hint that she has a set ambition in medicine. This conclusion also provided an easy segue into her sales pitch. The interviewer may naturally respond by asking, "So what is your ambition in medicine?" This is a great example of subtly driving the conversation toward topics you wish to discuss (anything related to your pitch).

Notice how Cheyenne's answer was brief and to-the-point. Although she is revealing pieces of her sales pitch in her response, she answers the question. Now the interviewer can choose which aspects of her response he wishes to hear more about. He may want to hear more about Ayurveda, about Cheyenne's relationship with her grandmother, or about how she plans to apply holistic approaches in her practice of medicine. Either way, because Cheyenne stuck to aspects of her sales pitch (an inspiration, an interest, and intro to her ambition) in her response, expanding on any of these topics is still within her sales pitch (and thus her comfort zone).

Example 2: Another question related to why you chose to go into medicine

INTERVIEWER:
The future of medicine looks bleak. Why do you want to go into it?

CHEYENNE:
I want to go into medicine because I don't agree with the opinion that the future of this art is bleak. I agree that there are problems in health-care delivery in America today; however, these are largely the result of complex political and social dynamics. Medical advances today are the most incredible they have ever been, and medical research is growing exponentially. I mentioned earlier that I see opportunities to improve Western medicine with more holistic approaches; I also hope to engage in policy change and program development to improve the practice of medicine. I see medicine as a growing and evolving field that will fulfill many of my interests.

Cheyenne did a great job here of balancing her response with information that addressed the question and information from her sales pitch. She showed the interviewer that she was aware of factors that may make medicine seem like a tough field to get into, but was confident in saying that she did not agree with this perception. She then provided support for her opinion that the future of medicine is not bleak. Interviewers like to see that you are willing to defend your beliefs with confidence and grace.

Cheyenne very tactfully dropped the hint that she views medicine as an art, and that she would like to get involved in public policy and programmatic aspects of health care. Of course, these are all aspects of her sales pitch. She concludes strongly with a nice lead-in to her sales pitch via her interests; you can see how it would be natural for the questioner to ask in response, "What are these interests that you feel medicine will fulfill and how?" This would allow Cheyenne to further elaborate on her sales pitch by discussing her various interests and motivations and how they lead into her ambition.

Another noteworthy aspect of this response is that she linked her response to this question to her last response (Example 1) by referring once again to her desire to incorporate holistic healing into her medical practice. By doing so, she reinforces what she was talking about (the interviewer is more likely to remember something you repeat) and she makes the interview seem more like a conversation. The more conversational your interview is, the easier it will be for you to weave in your sales pitch. Furthermore, the sales pitch seems more unified if you can tie the pieces together in this subtle manner.

Example 3: Still another question related to why you chose to go into medicine

> INTERVIEWER:
> Describe what you believe to be the financial rewards of medicine.
>
> CHEYENNE:
> Well, I think it's pretty rewarding that I can earn a living doing work I enjoy. I actually hope to work abroad, so for me a career in medicine is also a passport that enables me to work anywhere in the world. Being able to experience different cultures and live internationally through my work is another rewarding aspect of a career in medicine.

Did you see how Cheyenne nicely diverted a potentially ugly question? Because money is a touchy subject (generally, money is not considered a good enough reason to go into medicine), she took the opportunity to discuss other rewards of medicine. Of course, the rewards she discussed came right out of her sales pitch (international travel). Notice the pattern here: every response contains some aspect of her sales pitch. This makes it natural for the interviewer to follow up by asking about the aspect of her sales pitch she mentioned. In this example, the interviewer may naturally want to ask about her ambitions abroad.

Example 4: Question related to why you will be a good doctor (because you have the ability to evaluate yourself and determine how you need to improve)

> INTERVIEWER:
> If you could change anything about yourself, what would it be?
>
> CHEYENNE:
> Well, I have a tendency to get bored quickly. That's part of the reason I was drawn to medicine, actually. I need to be in a field that is constantly evolving—with infectious diseases, I know I will be continually learning and adapting my practice. Similarly, by engaging myself in public health activities, I get to interface with communities in more than just a clinical manner. This, and aspiring to an international career, will keep me adapting my practice of medicine. I realize that to get there I will also have to be patient and accept things in their own time, so I'm working on that now.

Cheyenne hadn't really included weaknesses in her sales pitch (and neither should you), but she could easily remember one of the weaknesses that she had listed in her self-reflection chart. She chose a weakness that is easily forgivable. You don't ever want to bring up a weakness that may seriously affect your candidacy. Again, she's delivering more and more of her sales pitch. She goes into more detail on why she is drawn to her chosen ambition and the subspecialties she wants to pursue. Cheyenne remembered our tip about how med schools love to see inward reflection, so she shows them that she understands how to admit a flaw and work on changing herself.

So don't talk about how you are a kleptomaniac or can't stand old people.

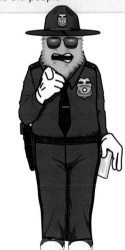

Example 5: Another question related to why you will be a good doctor

> INTERVIEWER:
> What do you do to alleviate stress?
>
> CHEYENNE:
> Art provides me with my stress relief! I talked about painting in my personal statement, but I also dance and perform spoken word. These aspects of my life are just as important to me as my professional activities; in Ayurveda, balance is one of the most important elements of good health. Similarly, from the perspective of holistic healing, one's mental health is a great determinant of one's physical health. In fact, this is also a topic central to my ambitions in medicine. As recent research shows, stress is an important modulator of immune function. In the future, I hope to incorporate stress reduction and nutrition therapy into HIV-care regimens.
>
> or
>
> Art provides me with my stress relief! I talked about painting in my personal statement, but I also perform spoken word and dance. Through samba, West African dance, and classical Indian dance, I have also been able to learn a lot about these respective cultures. Although I've travelled to Brazil and India, I have yet to visit Africa. I mentioned before that I look forward to working abroad; my ambition is to work in international HIV/AIDS, and I'm hoping to spend some time living in Africa.

In this example, we provided two possible responses to demonstrate that it doesn't really matter what aspects of your sales pitch you touch on. What's important is that you *do* touch on some part of it in your responses. In her first response, Cheyenne answers the question and then transitions into her ambition by talking about holistic healing (reinforced again!). In the second, she discusses her extracurricular interests (dance and travel) in order to transition into her ambition. The most important thing is that she directs the conversation to her desired topic. In both responses, Cheyenne concludes by revealing her ambition in medicine.

Example 6: Question intended to see how you react to stress

> INTERVIEWER:
> Tell me all you know about protein folding.
>
> CHEYENNE:
> Okay. There are four levels of protein structure. The primary structure of a protein is its amino acid sequence…etc….etc…

Surprise! Not every question has to lead into your sales pitch. You don't want to appear too contrived. If a question really does not have much to do with your sales pitch, you can just answer the question. On the other hand, if Cheyenne had envisioned a future in proteonomics, this question would have been a great opportunity to go into her ambitions.

6.4 Should I Be Doing Anything Else to Prepare?

There are a lot of pretty ridiculous suggestions out there about how to prepare for interviews. Some of the most infamous ones, and their relative merits, are discussed below:

Read the Newspaper Everyday

If you already do this, that's great. However, most premeds are super busy and barely have time to eat, much less stay informed on world events. A more realistic option is to set up your email homepage to include a news ticker; most email providers have this option. That way when you are logging onto your account, you can skim the headlines that are most popular, and spend a few minutes browsing articles you find interesting. Alternatively, there are several internet news services that offer free updates (e.g. www.oneworld.net) that you can customize by topic. It's rare to be asked about current events, and even if you don't know the answer to a question about recent news, this isn't going to keep you out of medical school. The most important aspect of the interview is conveying that you will be a good medical student. If your interviewer wishes to discuss a current event that you are not familiar with, simply admit it and ask the interviewer for a bit of background on the topic.

Try to Sketch Out Your Answers To One Of Those Lists Of 1000 Interview Questions

These lists are good for giving you an idea of the huge breadth of possible questions that may arise in an interview. From what we've heard, *anything* can happen in an interview; there is no guarantee that your memorizing answers to a huge list of questions will prepare you for an interview. Plus, it's a huge time sink. You'll realize that the important questions in the interview should all be answerable from your sales pitch and self-reflection chart. You *know* this stuff, after all, as its all about you. If you happen to come across a list of sample interview questions, use it to see how you can lead into your sales pitch while answering each question.

Keep up on all the latest advances in medicine

Yeah right! How about a more feasible goal? Do a search for recent developments related to the ambition you picked for your sales pitch. This could be a quick internet search, or require pulling a few journal articles. Either way, by narrowing your scope to latest advances related to your ambition, the task becomes one you can accomplish in half an hour. More importantly, should the subject of medical advances/recent research arise, you're discussion will be consistent with your sales pitch.

Practice in front of a mirror

Sure, why not. It won't hurt you to practice your pitch in front of the mirror, but it isn't the best way to work on your public-speaking skills. It is actually much more helpful to practice with a friend, or family member. A mirror won't give your feedback. Key things include the volume of your speech, the speed at which you speak, eye contact, and how often you use placeholders in your speech (e.g. "umm," "like," "you know what I mean," "or whatever").

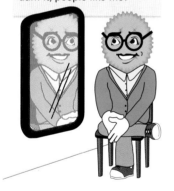

Because I'm smart enough, I'm good enough, and gosh darn it, people like me!

6.5 Tips for Success

In addition to our suggestions above, here are some realistic tips on how to prepare for your interviews.

6.5.1 Getting into the Right Mindset

This may be the most difficult part of preparing for interviews. Interviewing is draining, repetitive, and nerve-racking. You will only survive this gracefully if you develop a core of confidence concerning your application. Hopefully, developing your sales pitch has helped you to develop this confidence. You now know exactly how to market yourself and that is huge! You already have a great advantage over other applicants who have made it this far. In addition, do whatever it takes to make yourself feel good before an interview, whether that means a mocha latte or a five mile run. At the very least, give yourself 10 minutes in the morning of every interview day to center yourself and refresh your motivation.

6.5.2 Group Interviews

Group interviews can be weird. You are in a room with a few other candidates, and that immediately makes the interview feel competitive. It's fascinating to watch how peoples' personalities change in a competitive environment. Unfortunately, it's really easy to see who gets super nervous, who turns into psycho premed narcissist, and who seems unphased by the competitive vibe. So, be cool. Don't worry about competition. It's possible that the four people in an interview group will all be accepted, and you need to go into the interview with that mindset. Treat your fellow interviewees as though they were your fellow med school classmates, meaning respectfully. This means allowing everyone to finish speaking, staying attentive, and contributing in a balanced way. If someone else in the group doesn't show these courtesies, it will just make you look better, so stay conscious of your manners. It helps if you reference other candidates' responses, so that the atmosphere has a flowing conversational feel; this will show that you are comfortable communicating in a group environment and are attentive to the other members' contributions.

Remember that you are being evaluated individually, not as a group, so your sales pitch is still key in this setting. It's unlikely that you will deliver your full pitch in a group interview. Your goals are to present relevant parts of your sales pitch in the context of your responses, and to exude comfort within a group setting. You may be asked questions to which anyone can choose to respond. Respond to questions that can lead into aspects of your sales pitch.

6.5.3 Multiple Interviews

Three to five interviews in one day is standard at most schools, and it's for your own benefit; this way you have more than one chance to make a good impression! Going over your sales pitch over and over again may seem repetitive, but it's best to be consistent. Remember that interviewers will submit summaries, or discuss in person, your application with others on the admissions committee. It's best to be consistent in your performance so that all of your interviewers walk away with the same impression. (See section 1.2.2 for more on how admissions committees work.) Yes, it will get redundant. But this is all part of the song and dance that is the admissions process.

6.5.4 Don't Let Your Guard Down!

During the interview run, you will interact with many other players in the admissions process. You may have breakfast with the admissions director, go on a tour with a current student, do paperwork with a secretary, be in a room with a group of applicants all day, etc. You must remain poised in all of these interactions. Anyone that interacts with you on interview day may have contact with the admissions committee. (Read our section 1.2.3 for a story demonstrating the importance of this concept.)

6.5.5 Follow Up

Following up with an interviewer is one of the easiest things to do, yet many applicants are too bogged down to do it. Get an advantage over your fellow applicants by writing thank you letters to your interviewers. You can compose a standard response, which you can customize appropriately. Interviewers will like to see you reference some aspect of your interview to make this gesture more personal. You may mail or email the notes to each interviewer individually, or send them all to the admissions office.

6.5.6 Appearance, Maintanance, and Logistics

Here is a table of some of the most common logistical issues during interview trips, and our suggestions for each one:

Common Issues	Our Suggested Prevention
Static Cling This is such a common problem that a few admissions secretaries have static-cling spray on hand. Dress socks and pantyhose are the most common culprits of static cling.	Keep static-cling dryer sheets in your wardrobe bag with your suit and in the compartment you pack your socks in. Alternatively, you could buy some anti-static spray (any store selling laundry supplies may carry this item) and keep some in a travel-size bottle.
Wrinkled Clothes It's not the end of the world if you have a huge diagonal crease in your suit jacket, but it does look about as tacky as not brushing your hair (Yes, you should groom your hair.)	Ask hotel staff, or the friend you are staying with, for their iron the night before your interview. If you don't have time to iron the night before, at least you won't be fumbling around in the dark at 6am trying to find an iron.
Snagged Pantyhose	Carry a spare pair.
Distracted by Hunger or a Sugar-crash Breakfast sessions are usually around 7am and lunch often doesn't come around until five hours later. Plus, you will be expending a lot of energy 'performing' all day long. If you are the type who eats throughout the day, you should keep some energizing snacks in your bag.	Granola bars and trail mix are portable and energy rich. You should avoid chocolate bars and sodas which may cause you to crash after your sugar high. Similarly, opting for the bagel instead of the cinnamon roll at breakfast may be a smarter idea. It's a good idea to carry some change for vending machines should you need gum, coffee, or pretzels at the last minute.

Forgotten Items Some of the most common include: Dress socks and pantyhose; underwear; pen and paper; breath fresheners; cash; travel tickets; ID; contact lens solution/case	Make a list of the items you should pack before your first interview. Go buy any travel items you don't have the week before your first interview. Just follow your checklist while packing for each trip. You may even want to keep a stash of interview travel items, so you don't have to think about them each trip.
Showing Up Late This is not tolerated by the medical institution at all. By and large, your medical school experience is going to involve high-level functioning at ungodly hours. The admissions staff have heard every excuse in the book and are jaded, so you really want to avoid being in this situation.	Plan for way more time than you think you need to get to your interview. Thirty minutes to an hour of buffer time is good. Parking may be far away from the admissions office; you may have to get gas or get lost; there could be a traffic jam. You get the idea. If you give yourself a buffer, you won't stress as much if something goes wrong on your way. If you arrive early, you have bonus time to center yourself and review your sales pitch, self-reflection chart, and your research on the school. Plus you'll make a good impression and avoid starting the day stressed out.

Figure 6.5.6 Appearance, Maintenance, and Logistics

6.6 WHAT IS INTERVIEW DAY LIKE?

6.6.1 The Structure of the Day

Breakfast

Interview days usually begin with an "Arrival of the Applicants" or similarly named breakfast event from anywhere between 7am and 9am. For these events, you should arrive near the beginning, even if it appears that you can arrive towards the end without incident. Studies show that a first impression of a person is formed within the first 30 seconds of meeting him or her and is difficult to change once established, so start off looking put-together and enthusiastic. Don't arrive at the breakfast half-dressed, expecting to sneak away to finish changing, grooming, etc. These breakfasts aren't very casual; they may be attended by faculty and admissions staff that register applicants upon arrival and make 'small-talk' rounds while you have coffee and bagels or whatever. As soon as you arrive, you should be on your best behavior—the entire day is part of the interview! Don't look at breakfast as a break; rather, treat it as a warm-up session. Your first awkward exchanges with other applicants at breakfast can be practice for a day full of talking to strangers about yourself and doing it with confidence and composure.

"Optional" Class/Tour/Admissions Presentation

Thankfully, few medical schools toss you into an interview right after breakfast. Most interviewers have to tend to their clinical duties in the early morning; however, some schools do schedule interviews as early as 8am. The post-registration slot is usually reserved for admissions and financial aid presentations, most commonly followed by an "optional" class visit (since lectures are sometimes only held in the morning). Sometimes tours are given in the morning, but more often these are scheduled around lunchtime or after interviews in the afternoon. Admissions and financial aid presentations are simple information-dissemination sessions. Thankfully, you can relax a little bit and just listen. It will be hard not to fall asleep, especially if they dim the lights for a PowerPoint presentation. So sit up straight, chew gum, or write notes—whatever it takes to stay awake.

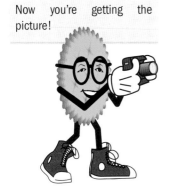
Now you're getting the picture!

For the "optional" class visit, think about whether you believe it's truly an optional activity. It may be tempting instead to take that extra coffee break or get a bit of shut-eye, and you should do this if you really need it. If the school has specifically arranged a class session for each applicant, don't miss it. Make sure to take note of who is lecturing and what class it is. If you choose not to go, prepare yourself for the possibility that your interviewers may ask you about your experience (what class you attended, who was lecturing, how you felt about it, and if you learned anything interesting). If you say you skipped out, you may risk seeming uninterested and lazy. Observing a class can be excruciatingly boring. You're the only one dressed in a suit and all the med students are checking you out. Meanwhile you don't have any context in which to place what they are teaching, but you have to look like you're interested. Plus, let's face it, basic science lectures generally aren't fun. If you don't have anything great to say about the experience, focus on some other compliment (e.g. how great the audiovisual equipment was or how comfortable the class size was).

As far as the tour goes, this is where you can have a little more flexibility. At the start of your interview circuit, you should go on a few tours to see what your setting will be like for the next four years. After a while, however, you'll start to realize that most hospitals look the same. Buildings will have different names, some will have colors, some won't, and some hospitals will be connected, others blocks apart. In any case, the informational yield of a tour decreases with each subsequent tour, and as an applicant, it's really difficult to assess what you're looking for in a facility. If you are stealthy, the tour, usually led by a student who only does tours, is the one thing that is relatively safe to skip. The student is almost always unaware of who is 'supposed to be' on the tour. If you are seriously interested in the school, though, the tour may be one of the most interesting and fun parts of the day. In short, go if you feel you'll get something out of it. Otherwise, use this time to recuperate and prepare for your next interview.

Lunch

Lunch isn't as monitored as the arrival breakfast, and it can be anything from a catered lunch in the admissions office to a complimentary lunch in the hospital cafeteria. The structure of the lunch session varies so you may be with a set group of people, or left to your own devices with a meal ticket. If you have pressing phone calls to make or something else to take care of, lunch is the safest time to do it. However, lunchtime also gives you a rare opportunity to talk to current medical students, and a wider variety of medical students will attend (free food for them).

Interviews

Most interviews will start after lunch, though some schools (e.g. Washington University) will have one interview after an orientation in the morning. The majority of medical schools will arrange for at least two to three interviews, more if you're an MD/PhD applicant. Your performance in the interviews is the most important part of your day. Don't be straggling behind everyone, don't be late, and don't count on time between interviews to collect yourself or use the restroom—do all that beforehand. If your interviews are stacked, your first interviewer will very likely escort you to your next interview. Carry around the folder you're given at the beginning of the day, but don't wear your coat or drag around a suitcase or backpack (briefcases, shoulder bags, and purses are okay). Most admissions offices have a coat closet where you may store your suitcase and coat. Try to avoid talking on your cell phone in the admissions office and keep it turned off in your bag; go outside during a break if you need to make a call.

The more comfortable you are with your sales pitch, the easier interviewing will be. Enjoy the interviews—it's hard for an interviewer to be terribly negative if you are enthusiastic and respectful. Remember that interviews are all about the three cardinal questions, and the three cardinal questions are all about *you!* You know yourself better than anyone, so the hardest part of the interview now is just maintaining your composure. We talk more about navigating tough questions in section 6.63 below.

Conclusion

At the end of the day, you will usually be asked by a member of the admissions staff to reconvene to fill out evaluations of your experience. Unless something egregious happened (like your interviewer made sexist comments), keep it positive and gracious. Evaluation forms are meant to be anonymous. Schools really do want to know if their interviewers are helping to convey a positive school image. We know of one applicant who was particularly upset by one of her interview experiences. From her vantage point, her interviewer flagrantly belittled her extracurricular experiences and concluded that she didn't have what it took to go to medical school. Feeling that the interviewer has crossed a boundary, she not only wrote a negative evaluation, but also sent a letter to the admissions office detailing what happened, hoping that interview could be excluded. As it turned out, the school had heard similar complaints, and the interviewer was unceremoniously booted from the admissions committee. The applicant was offered a letter of acceptance. Complaints should be justified and formally presented in writing. Only file a complaint if you have an inappropriate interaction during an interview that either you don't want someone else to experience or that may hurt your candidacy. Don't whine to admissions staff because you feel that you didn't prepare or perform as well as you could have.

Minority Student Gatherings

If you self-identified as an underrepresented minority applicant, you may be compelled to attend minority recruitment events. You may have a whole weekend of events or simply receive a packet of handouts, as minority recruitment varies greatly among schools. If you happen to be the only minority applicant on a particular day, you may receive a considerable amount of extra attention. Most schools, however, will simply have a gathering at the end of the day at which minority students can answer questions specific to their concerns. These sessions are a great way to get feedback on the lifestyle and experience of that community. Keep in mind that the minority students hosting these events will likely be *asked directly* about what they think of you. Some of these students might be voting committee members, so don't say anything you wouldn't want getting back to the admissions committee. The main reason admissions would follow up on you in this way is to determine whether you are sincerely interested in attending their school. Schools use valuable resources to recruit minority applicants, so they want to assess the probability that their investment will pay off. Some minority student hosts may be voting committee members, so making a positive impression is a plus.

6.6.2   Take Notes!

We know you don't want to look like a nerd, scribbling away all day. But, ave one blank sheet of paper with you to write down a few key phrases from each interview. This will help you to customize your follow-up letters, as well as to remember your experience. For example, if the Cornell interviewer provided Cheyenne with information on the school's extensive study abroad options (see **Figure 6.26a**), she could thank him for this in her follow-up and use this information to help choose between schools. It is also helpful to get each interviewer's business card. A great way to set up your note-taking is to fold your one piece of paper in half-lengthwise, taping business cards to one side and brief notes on your interaction on the other. On the reverse side, use one column for things you like, and the other for aspects of the school you aren't thrilled with. Don't walk around carrying a paper with "Things I Hate about this School" as a column heading! You should designate the columns in your mind and then just list general phrases (e.g. financial aid, hospital-record system, city). This way, only you know which aspects of the school you have designated as pluses or minuses. These one-pagers on the schools will be really helpful when you try to decide between schools.

6.6.3   Expect Tough Questions

Tough questions are a part of the interview experience. The schools are trying to decide between hundreds of qualified applicants, so seeing how you function under pressure is another way to evaluate you. As we mentioned earlier, doctors are expected to keep their cool under pressure. So just relax when faced with a tough question, because keeping your composure is the best way to respond.

In general, tough questions deal with ethical issues and are intended to stump you or directly challenge you. You saw how Cheyenne handled direct challenges in Example 2 above, and an indirect challenge in Example 4. Asking about a personal weakness or highlighting a flaw in your application are common ways in which interviewers challenge applicants. So be prepared to explain a low MCAT score or a C in organic chemistry by being mature enough to admit your mistakes and showing how you grew from the experience.

Other times, questions may be tough because they are 'traps.' In Examples 1 and 3 above, the interviewer asked his questions in a manner that made it easy for Cheyenne to fall into the trap of saying she was going into medicine because her family expects her to, or because she wants to make a lot of money. Cheyenne avoided these traps by staying focused on her sales pitch. Below we'll see how she calmly responds to a few ethical questions and being stumped.

Example 7: A Tough Ethical Question

INTERVIEWER:
Do you think it's ethical to use a fetus to harvest a cell line in order to save the life of a sibling with cancer?

CHEYENNE:
Well, this is a tough question for me to answer because I have mixed feelings on the topic. On one hand, stem cell therapies represent a great advance in our ability to save a cancer patient's life. On the other hand, we have to question whether it is just to sacrifice the life of the fetus.

According to my personal belief system, the final decision on whether this therapy is ethical should be up to the family. Medicine has this therapeutic option available, and it is the family's choice to use it or not, depending on their personal ethics. However, I recognize that a case-by-case analysis is not always feasible and as a society we have to set ethical standards. Interestingly, in my work abroad, I've realized that a society's ethics fluctuate with their cultural values, and thus what is ethical in one society may not be in another. For this reason, I support the establishment of committees to set guidelines for these kinds of ethical issues.

Cheyenne started off her response with a fantastic tactic: take a neutral stance. It's always safe to explore the two sides of a given issue. If you can identify with an aspect of each side, as Cheyenne did, you may even be viewed as more empathetic and open-minded than if you took a firm stance on one side of an issue. Keep in mind, however, that if you do have firm beliefs on an ethical issue, you should express them! You have to be yourself. Pretend you were discussing the given topic with a good friend: express your views and respect others' views in a balanced, non-confrontational manner. Cheyenne shows her confidence by frankly discussing her personal beliefs on the issue, even though her outlook may be unconventional. She then brings her response back to neutral ground by talking about ethical committees. Notice how she managed to weave in a little bit of her sales pitch with the comment on her experience.

Want to see it again? Here she repeats her performance with another question:

Example 8: Another Ethics Question

INTERVIEWER:
Should physicians be forced to treat patients?

CHEYENNE:
Again, I can relate to aspects on both sides of this issue. On one hand, if a physician is withholding care that could save someone's life, it seems to be a societal wrong. On the other hand, we have to question whether anyone should be forced to provide their services to help another.

Personally, I do not feel physicians should be forced to treat patients and this stems from my background. In my culture, death is an accepted part of the cycle of life, and similar to a DNR, I feel that patients should have the right to refuse treatment as part of their acceptance of death. Furthermore, in Ayurveda, the physician brings healing to the patient just as much with her intention as with her physical treatment. If a doctor does not want to treat a patient, the treatment will lack the intention of healing. To me, treatment without intention is a disservice to the patient.

I realize, however, that this ethical issue may have many contexts. A doctor could have various reasons for refusing treatment, and I think these cases should be reviewed on an individual basis. Perhaps doctors should only be obligated to find another physician to treat the patient if they refuse treating the patient themselves.

Again, Ms. Starr starts out neutralizing the issue by relating to both sides. She then conveys her personal opinion and drops in some of her sales pitch while doing so (reinforces her theme of holistic healing). If she didn't have a set stance on this topic, Cheyenne could have just begun her response with what she said in the third paragraph above, remaining on neutral ground.

Keep in mind that you don't have to be formulaic in your answers. We repeated a similar response in Examples 7 and 8 to show that the same tool can be used to answer any ethical question.

Example 9: Taking a Firm Stance on a Tough Ethics Question

> INTERVIEWER:
> What if a patient who is a Jehovah's Witness refuses surgery that is necessary to save his life? What would you do?
>
> CHEYENNE:
> I would respect his wishes. As I mentioned earlier, one's beliefs on life and death are a reflection of cultural values. I would not force anyone to undergo treatment.

Here is an example of taking a firm stance on a topic. Cheyenne didn't bother to teeter on the neutral side in this answer because she had a personal opinion on this topic already. Don't be afraid to speak your mind. Just as Cheyenne does, support your opinion (and try to be succinct). Remember to be respectful of other views on the subject while you are responding. For example, if you are against abortion, you can express this respectfully by saying, "My personal beliefs do not support the practice of abortion." You remain respectful by avoiding sweeping generalizations and harsh words such as, "I think the women who get abortions are killing their babies, and I don't support that." In general, it's socially acceptable to have a personal belief system that governs your actions, but unacceptable and condescending to impose your belief system on others.

Example 10: A Stumper Tough Question

> INTERVIEWER:
> Name four non–Arabic-speaking countries in the Middle East.
>
> CHEYENNE:
> I'm sorry; I don't know the answer to that question. However, I can research the answer and get back to you.

Yes, you can say "I don't know"! Obviously, it's not necessary for Cheyenne to know the answer to this question in order to be a good medical student. The point of a stumper is to catch you off-guard and make you nervous. Then interviewers want to see if you can admit that you don't know something. You'll look worse if you start making up an answer. If you know part of the answer to a question, then just say whatever part you know. Interviewers will appreciate it if you are willing to take the initiative and learn and report back to them. Just don't forget to do it! A great way to report back is in your follow-up note to them.

We've heard of candidates being asked inappropriate questions, but just thinking of them as part of the expected 'tough questions' during the interview. This is not true. As aforementioned, inappropriate questions are unfortunately common in the interview process. (Perhaps this is because many interviewers are volunteers without any formal training on how to interview.) Interviewers have been known to ask questions about marriage, having kids, spouses, and even sexual orientation. Questions that may seem to discriminate against race, gender, age, or sexual orientation are not appropriate. How applicants handle these questions can vary from one individual to the next. Some applicants may not have a problem discussing why they got divorced, while others would rather crawl into a hole than discuss their personal relationships in a medical school interview. If you don't feel a question is appropriate, just say that you don't feel comfortable answering and ask nicely to move on to the next question. You can always also ask tactfully how such a question is relevant to the interview. **Most importantly, only answer a question if you feel comfortable doing so**.

6.7 NON-TRADITIONAL APPLICANTS

For the most part, older applicants are viewed by medical schools as assets; they have less concern that you will show up to clinic hungover or call in sick after dancing the night away. However, if you are getting into your 30s and 40s, your stamina and family obligations will be topics difficult to avoid during interviews. Instead, you should strive to emphasize a record of solid, upwardly mobile career progressions and achievements, and show medical schools that you have the stamina for a challenging career in medicine, whatever your age. Ultimately, age is just one variable in the highly complex equation of medical school admissions. In the 2005 application season, the oldest matriculating student nationwide was 53, so anything is possible.

Our advice is to realize that you are not alone. There are thousands of non-traditional applicants each year, all with different stories, and they make it through medical school just fine. You won't be the first student to have a baby during medical school, or to possibly lose a parent (two issues that interviewers tend to ask about with older applicants). And you should relate this to your questioner, demonstrating the maturity that will help you through these situations should they arise. After all, older applicants may be more likely to have a baby during school, but they are also more likely to have the time-management skills and focus to be able to handle a newborn during the next four years.

Technically, admissions committees should not discriminate on the basis of age, marital status, or other social criteria; however, this information tends to seep into the decision process. So if you are the struggling single father of three toddlers, or a single woman whose maternal clock is ticking, you don't want to emphasize those issues.

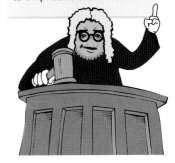

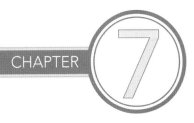
INTERVIEW BLOOPERS: ENCOURAGEMENT

7.1 MURPHY'S LAW

Unfortunately, Murphy's Law and the principles of entropy are very likely to influence your time on the interview trail. When it does happen, don't worry or get flustered; trust us, it happens to the best of applicants. No matter how prepared you are when you arrive or how early you begin travelling to your interviews, something will inevitably go wrong. Fortunately, for most people, this might mean something as mundane as stepping in mud on the sidewalk, breaking a heel, or forgetting an umbrella. We hope you don't have to deal with anything more serious. We've included a few (true!) interview-day blooper stories which may be of help or comfort to you should you have the misfortune of experiencing something embarrassing or just plain awful. Rest assured that the applicants in these stories ended up ultimately being admitted to top-ten institutions, sometimes to the very schools at which the bloopers occurred! Most importantly, these applicants were successful because they turned these bloopers into learning experiences.

7.2 Airline Mishap

Okay, so this applicant cut things a *little* close. This particular applicant, whom we'll call Frank, arranged to fly in January, to an interview at the University of Chicago on an early-morning flight from the East Coast. Fortunately for Frank, Chicago's infamous weather, normally a hazy, snowy blur that time of year, was actually clear and calm. Frank boarded his flight on time at 5:30am in Boston and was scheduled to land at Chicago's Midway Airport at 8:15am, leaving him only 45 minutes to get to his interview on time. He figured that was okay since the cab ride to the University of Chicago's medical school was only ten minutes from this airport.

The flight took off on time with everything going as planned, including Frank's sleep 'catch-up.' Forty-five minutes prior to landing, the captain announced that there was a medical emergency on board the aircraft. Crap! Frank, as a mere applicant, lacked any qualifications to assist in the situation, and, a diverted flight would devastate his interview-day schedule. Crap, Crap! Cell phones don't work at 30,000 feet. The captain made an announcement: the aircraft would be diverted to Cleveland to deal with the emergency and would then continue on to Chicago O'Hare, a massive airport located over an hour from UChicago.

Unable to control the situation, Frank arrived at Chicago O'Hare at 10:00am and called UChicago as soon as he landed. The secretary seemed sympathetic and told him to come as soon as possible. Frank arrived at around 10:45am, and the secretary even reimbursed his cab fare. Unfortunately, the incident dominated his interactions for the rest of the day. Every interview started with, "Oh, you're the one that was on the diverted flight…" One interviewer asked him outright why he didn't fly in the night before, as most applicants did. (Ouch!) Even though the incident wasn't his fault, Frank ended up looking irresponsible. He didn't end up going to UChicago, but he learned an important lesson about allowing time for the unexpected in his interview arrangements. Retrospectively, Frank recognized that he was on the defensive for most of the day and tried to avoid the subject when interviewers brought it up. He realized that he could have turned the incident into an opportunity to lead into his sales pitch and kept a positive attitude or a sense of humor about the situation. (For example, he could have responded by saying, "Funny enough, all I could think about besides the possibility of missing my interviews was how helpless I felt. I'm really looking forward to the day where I have the knowledge and skills to help people no matter where I am!). Learning these two lessons helped him succeed in his subsequent interviews, and he ended up at a top-five institution. Don't let being flustered over an unexpected event sabotage your interviews! If something beyond your control happens, try to see how you can use the incident as an opportunity to lead into your sales pitch!

7.3 AIRLINE TIA (TRANSIENT ISCHEMIC ATTACK—MEDICAL SPEAK FOR ZONING OUT)

Another applicant, whose name shall not be revealed, had just finished a three-day MD/PhD interview at Washington University, and had just one day to get to his next interview for the MD program at Penn. This applicant was exhausted after three days of interviews, student dinners, orientation meetings, and tours, and arrived at the airport at less than full energetic capacity. When he arrived at the airport, he realized that weather delays had thrown St Louis airport timetables into disarray; many flights were delayed or cancelled. His original flight was delayed, so he took a little nap.

When he woke up, he went to the boarding gate for his flight to Philadelphia, handed his boarding card to the agent, got on the flight, and fell asleep. When he woke up again, he heard an announcement that said "Ladies and gentlemen, we are beginning our final approach into George Bush International Airport…" The applicant thought, "Oh, I guess the name of Philadelphia's airport changed because of the election," and returned to his restful slumber. Upon disembarking the plane, an overly helpful Continental Airlines employee welcomed him to Houston, jolting the applicant. "What?! This is Houston?" he asked desparately, startling the Continental Airlines staff. The staff member, after learning the applicant was supposed to board another carrier's flight to Philadelphia, was baffled as to how the applicant was allowed to board a completely different carrier to a totally different destination. After taking the applicant to the ticket counter, a brief, yet heated, discussion ensued over who was responsible for getting the applicant to Philadelphia.

Thankfully, the airline accepted the applicant's argument that bore some responsibility for ensuring that passengers boarded their flights. However, the applicant still needed to make a phone call, as he was going to be arriving late to his interview at Penn. The apologetic applicant told the truth, gave the admissions staff some comic relief, and rescheduled for later in the week. Despite his lapse in judgment, he was eventually admitted to Penn.

The applicant learned to make sure he got enough sleep, and this meant shifting his 'night-owl' sleep-wake pattern to match the demands of interviews, which require early-morning performance. He also learned to avoid scheduling back-to-back interviews in different cities!

7.4 FOOT-IN-MOUTH

A minority applicant, whom we'll call Tyrone, made the mistake of letting his guard down at a conservative institution. As this was his first interview, he set out to impress Cornell Medical School with his familiarity with the school and the uniqueness of his career goals. However, Tyrone had never been to Cornell and was a little thrown off by the atmosphere and location of the school. He expected that any school in Manhattan would thrive on the diversity that is the hallmark of the city. To his great surprise, Cornell seemed to be a reflection of the wealthy, conservative, and Caucasian Upper East Side neighborhood which surrounded the school. Minority students and staff seemed to be scarce on interview day, though admissions had arranged for a few minority students to meet with him at the end of the day.

Tyrone's first interviewer, after a great, vibrant discussion, took him on a personal tour of one of the hospitals, which is not a common occurrence during medical school interviews. Having established a seemingly casual and candid report with the interviewer, Tyrone let down his guard. Halfway through the tour, Tyrone joked, "Wow, not too many underserved patients here, huh?" His sixty-something Caucasian interviewer seemed a little taken aback but continued the tour. Tyrone knew he flubbed based on his interviewer's reaction, and was more restrained in the second interview and during subsequent events. However, he ended up looking immature and unable to draw the line concerning what comments are appropriate in a given situation—not really a good fit with the ideal of doctors being societal role models.

Unfortunately, Tyrone was not admitted to Cornell, though he doesn't know if it was because of his little slip. Most importantly, Tyrone learned from his first interview experience that everything he says and does during interview day may affect his evaluation. He made a concerted effort to be more professional in his later interviews and was eventually admitted to four schools, two of which were top-fives. If Tyrone were really set on Cornell, he could have sought out the interviewer and apologized for his flippant question. Although apologizing for a blooper may not make it disappear, it only helps to show your maturity and sense of self-awareness.

7.5 WHERE ARE MY SHOES?

Constant travel begins to take its toll on even the most seasoned travellers. Additionally, the more one travels, the more likely something is to go wrong, which is what happened to one poor applicant, whom we'll call Ally. Ally turned in her AMCAS application a *wee* bit after the recommended submission date (early September), but fortunately, she was a very competitive applicant. She was able to secure interviews at almost every school to which she applied, but because of first-come-first-serve scheduling, her interviews had to be stacked in a whirlwind rush in January and early February. So, Ally flies to California for a couple of interviews and then flies back to New York for an interview at Columbia. When Ally arrives at New York's Kennedy airport, she patiently awaits her luggage to return on the carousel… and waits… then waits some more. It doesn't arrive! Ally specifically flew to New York the night before her interview to get a good night's sleep and be on time for her interview at Columbia, but her clothes were somewhere else! Luckily, the female friend with whom Ally was staying was a similar size and was able to lend her some clothes. However, their shoe sizes were different, and Ally's heels were in her checked luggage. Ally went to bed that night praying the airline would somehow manage to deliver her bag by 7am so that she would have professional shoes to wear to the interview.

7am arrived and went, and Ally really needed to get on the subway to Washington Heights- no word from the airline regarding her luggage. She briefly wandered a couple of streets to see if a shoe shop might be open; no such luck. Contemplating the situation, Ally decided it was best not to risk being late. So she turned up to the breakfast on time, in a nice suit, but with fairly ratty sneakers on. Although nobody asked about the sneakers outright, if she saw an interviewer's gaze shift to her feet she would briefly mention that her luggage got lost. By showing up on time and not treating her sneakers as a big deal, she showed her maturity in prioritizing what is important. In this manner, she let a potential disaster seem like no big deal. Ally focused on her sales pitch, had a few laughs over the sneakers throughout the day, and three months later, she received a fat acceptance package from Columbia.

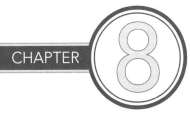

ONCE YOU START HEARING FROM SCHOOLS

8.1 HOW LONG SHOULD I WAIT BEFORE SAYING YES?

If you received one or more offers, congratulations! In 2005, seven thousand five hundred and fifty lucky applicants received multiple acceptances (approximately 39% of all accepted applicants). They will face a dilemma that is the envy of tens of thousands of applicants across the country. Most schools will let you know at the beginning of March if they are going to offer you a place in their incoming class. You are permitted to hold multiple acceptances until May 15th of the year following your application. After May 15th, you should hold only one spot, though you may remain on waitlists until you matriculate. If you started the process on time, you'll have around two months to attend second-look weekends at the schools in which you are truly interested (unless you are a minority or MD/PhD applicant, expenses are typically your responsibility). These second-look weekends will be more relaxed than your interview visits as the pressure to get accepted will be gone. On your second visit, you are free to voice any reservations or considerations you have in making your choice with current students and faculty, who may provide valuable information for your decision.

But still avoid getting plastered at the wine-and-cheese mixer.

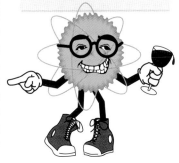

Take your time. Four years is a long time, and medical school won't always be the most enjoyable experience. This is your time to make as informed a decision as possible about the environment, people, and facilities you will be frequenting both when you're having fun and when all you want to do is get ten more minutes of precious sleep. From March onward, depending on when you are accepted, is the period when you reflect back on what you truly value in a medical school. Refer back to the research and one-pagers you did during Phases 1-3 of the admissions process. If you have new ambitions or concerns, now is the time to look into those facets of the school.

Another factor you will probably need to take into consideration is financial aid. Sometimes, you will receive an offer of acceptance and need to wait on a financial-aid offer. If this is the case, it is considered acceptable to hold onto multiple acceptances for a prolonged period of time (until May 15th); otherwise, the AAMC 'recommends' students withdraw from schools as soon as they know they do not intend to matriculate (to be fair to other applicants). If you have multiple acceptances, you will receive multiple aid offers. Despite the fact that aid is 'need'-based, your package could vary wildly depending on the relative wealth of the school. Cash-strapped schools are very likely to ask you to contribute more, and offer you high-interest private loans; wealthier schools will most likely be more generous with scholarships. Once you receive your packages, refer to section 8.3 for suggestions on how to proceed.

It probably goes without saying that once you begin orientation at a medical school, it is generally not advisable to remain on waitlists at other institutions or hold other offers of acceptance. Our advice is to play it safe, but be persistent in pursuing what you want.

8.2 Do I Have Any Hope on the Waitlist?

The waitlist is actually a pretty good place to be! However, sitting by the phone or near the mailbox is not the way to be proactive here. First, you need to understand the typical organization of waitlists, and second, learn some ways to wow admissions committees into admitting you.

Waitlists are tiered at many medical schools. Some of these schools automatically tell you on which tier waitlist you are listed; others will give you this information only if you ask for it. If your letter says that you are in the first tier (particularly if it indicates that you are at the top of the first tier), you are in good shape. After May 15th, the high-flyer applicants holding 10 acceptances will have to eventually concede nine of them. Imagine this scenario occurring many times over many schools, and you can imagine the number of spots that open up at the end of May and the beginning of June. Medical schools often utilize waitlists to 'hip-pocket' applicants whom they filed as 'maybe' after the interview round. Either your application wasn't considered competitive enough, or they didn't think you were likely to choose their institution. This is why taking proactive measures is important—it's worth 'fighting' for an acceptance off of the waitlist at a school you really want to attend. Whether a waitlist is tiered or ranked does not change the fact that certain applicants will stand out among the rest. Your goal is to be one of these applicants.

What proactive measures can you take to stand out? Well, you get to be a little creative in this process, but there are some bread-and-butter moves that you can make to help alleviate the waitlist lull. If you are on a waitlist for your top-choice school, you must send a first-choice letter. A letter addressed to the director of admissions indicating why that particular school is your first choice is an effective tool to address the school's concern that you wouldn't accept an offer. But be warned: don't send multiple first-choice letters. The AAMC maintains a list of the schools you have applied to and to which you have been accepted. All medical schools have access to this information. Admissions directors between schools of a similar tier (e.g. Harvard & Stanford, Vanderbilt & Jefferson) tend to communicate frequently, particularly during waitlist time. If you casually come up in discussion just after both directors received a first-choice letter from you, you can be sure you aren't getting into either school. Medicine is, for better or for worse, a fairly small and chatty community, and you should always act under the assumption that word will get around.

Now you have to address the second possibility—that your application wasn't as competitive as you'd hoped. You need to remind the school of why you are a great candidate, and you have great creative license with which to do so. Feel free to think outside the box, keeping the following things in mind: your goal is to reemphasize why you would make an excellent medical student and physician, why you want to attend that school, and why you are just *so* unique and interesting that they would be foolish to exclude you from their incoming class. One waitlisted applicant we know created an album of why he was a great candidate. He included letters from family and friends extolling various qualities and photographs of himself engaged in extracurricular activities and lab work, and he put it all together with a sense of humor. Not only was the applicant memorable, but he also got in. Whether it was his spunk, his guts, or the quality of the album that earned him an acceptance, he doesn't know. Just remember that admissions committees are human, and running through this whole routine year after year has got to be tough; so you can imagine that a creative endeavour is refreshing for them. We're not saying to run off to the photo lab to get snap shot developed to ship off to medical schools, but if you can think of a creative way to support your application, go for it. Another candidate we know incorporated her first-choice letter and sales pitch into a poem (she also got accepted). At the very least, admissions committees will appreciate your effort!

If you are not in touch with your creative side, don't worry. You may choose to support your application with a simple letter detailing some of your recent achievements or activities. Through a discussion of your recent activities, you can highlight aspects of your sales pitch. If you choose to right a letter, it's a good idea to combine this with your first-choice letter. This way you talk about both why you are great and why you should be at that particular school in one shot. All of this information is straight from your sales pitch, self-reflection chart, and Researching Schools III (**Chapter 6**).

8.3 Deferring Admission

After you have received an acceptance, many schools offer the option of deferring entry to the following school year. The deferral option was created for students whose personal circumstances change between applying and receiving an acceptance, so that they can avoid having to go through the process again. However, there are a sizeable number of schools that grant deferrals more liberally, so more students are taking advantage of the deferral option to take a year off before matriculating.

If you are considering a deferral, you should check the policies of schools to which you were admitted to ascertain the feasibility of requesting and being granted a deferral. Schools will not entertain a deferral request until you have accepted a position in their incoming class by submitting a deposit. Many of the top institutions will grant deferrals fairly liberally as a rule of thumb, and the less competitive institutions will tend to be more rigid as they strain to fill their incoming classes. Even for schools that are more generous with deferrals, you will need to write an approximately one-page statement on the reason for requesting the deferral. If the deferral is granted, you are 'conditionally' guaranteed a spot in the following year's matriculating class. The conditions stipulated could be as simple as providing a brief update on what you've accomplished during your deferral year. As long as you are able to demonstrate that you've done something tangible and advantageous your personal and professional growth and have sorted out whatever problem you may have indicated as a reason to defer, the medical school should honor your deferred acceptance offer.

8.4 FINANCIAL AID PACKAGES

Either with your offer or shortly thereafter (if you filed your Free Application for Federal Student Aid, or FAFSA, and institution-specific financial aid forms on time), you should receive a financial aid offer. A typical offer consists of scholarship money, federal educational (Stafford) loans, private loans, and expected family/student contributions. Some schools, especially state schools and Caribbean schools, will not give scholarship money, but most will. You most likely won't have to begin paying back loans until after residency, but you need to make sure that your aid package is reasonable for you now. Here are a few pointers on evaluating financial aid offers:

Scholarships and Grants

Are there other scholarships or grants that you can qualify for? Oftentimes, financial aid offices have a list of resources for additional funding. Your scholarships and grants are usually awarded based on the activity and interests sheets that the financial aid offices ask you to fill out. One of the biggest mistakes applicants make is to neglect to submit this form. We know you are burnt out from AMCAS, but the more detail you provide in these forms, the more likely you are to match scholarship criteria.

Federal Loans

Check out how much of your Stafford loans are subsidized versus unsubsidized. The difference is that the government pays the interest on your subsidized loans from the time they are disbursed to the time you begin repayment. But you pay all of the interest on an unsubsidized Stafford. The government contracts out to many different lending institutions (e.g. Wells Fargo Bank, Sallie Mae) that service your loan. You get to choose the lender through which you want to receive your Stafford loans. Look for lenders that don't charge any origination fees. Oftentimes the lenders charge fees, so ask your financial aid office about the fees charged by their suggested Stafford lender.

Private Loans

Find out what the interest rates and repayment options are for all of your private loans! Many institutions will offer private loans, and they can set their own rules, so private loans don't have any set standard. For this reason, they often have really high interest rates and stringent repayment options. You may find that you can get a better educational loan from your bank. Many banks offer specialized loans for education, and even medical education specifically. If your credit isn't great, these private loans may be your best option.

Expected Family Contribution (EFC)

This is a weird component of your application, because it relies on your parents' financial information. You may have been independent for many years, or be 50 years old, and they will still ask for your parents' financial information to assess the EFC! If this number, which is generated by FAFSA, is really misrepresentative, write a letter to your financial aid office. Explain to them why your EFC is too high, and see if they can work with you on that figure. Typically, schools take the EFC from FAFSA and subtract that from their estimated attendance costs to calculate your "unmet financial need." It is this unmet-need figure that is used to determine how much you get in scholarships and loans. So you can see how much it may affect you if your EFC is not reflective of your family's true ability to contribute.

If financial aid is the only thing holding you back from attending your favorite school, communicate with them. You should be up front with schools about your aid package and your ability to pay. Sometimes, some extra money may emerge that could be incorporated into your package.

8.4 Leveraging Offers

It's difficult when you get a better aid offer from a school you don't want to attend as much. If you find yourself in this situation, and the aid package at your school of choice isn't going to ruin you financially, go to the school you prefer. After all, if you are like the average medical student and about to take on tens of thousands of dollars in educational debt, a fraction of that is not worth sacrificing the school of your choice. On the other hand, if the financial aid package is really making or breaking your decision, talk to the admissions director at your top choice. Remember, schools that accept you, particularly if they number more than two, are keen to have you matriculate. They already know which schools you hold acceptances to, so talking about another offer is not taboo. You can respectfully present the situation, letting them know that your aid package is the only thing holding you back from accepting their offer. Before contacting the director, however, have your aid information on hand, as they will want to discuss your other aid packages and the amount of additional aid you are looking for from their school. What they'll typically ask is:

- How much in scholarships are the other schools offering?
- What amount would you need for money to cease being an issue in your decision to accept?

You should be honest with schools about your other offers; as we said earlier, they will probably call up those schools to confirm the details. Honesty can pay off. One applicant a few years ago received acceptances to both Duke and Johns Hopkins. He really wanted to attend Hopkins, but Hopkins gave him less scholarship money. After Hopkins called to ask about his decision, he voiced his concerns about aid; all of a sudden, he was telling them how much Duke was offering, and Hopkins replied, "we'll see what we can do." Two days later, a FedEx package arrived at his home from Hopkins, offering him a scholarship worth $2,000 more than Duke's. In addition, often financial aid offers made later in the acceptance cycle are smaller as the more cash-strapped schools exhaust their budgets fairly quickly, so it's to your advantage to apply early.

8.5 RESEARCHING SCHOOLS IV

At this point, how do you pick the right school? Or more importantly, what should you be looking for in a school that will be important to your future success? Don't forget, the question you are asking yourself is where you will be happiest and most successful. So, as we mentioned earlier, refer back to your research from the interview phase (**Chapter 6**, Section Researching Schools III) In addition, you may want to use the following criteria to compare schools:

8.5.1 Curriculum
Examine the curricula of your schools carefully. You've probably already done this to some extent, but at this juncture you should evaluate in which curriculum you would work best and which

would prepare you best for clinics and residency. For example, if you're not a big lecture person, you might run into a lot of trouble at Cornell, where there are mandatory quizzes and problem-based learning sessions every week. Conversely, if you were an English major who barely remembers biology, you might want a hand-holding two year basic science curriculum before being tossed into the subjective and sporadically supervised world of clinics. Look at not only the amount of clinical exposure you would get in the first two years, but also what your day-to-day schedule would be like. Some schools have lecture from 9am-5pm, while others finish lectures around 2pm everyday!

8.5.2   The Boards

This is one of those things you don't really want to think about when you're applying and doing second-looks, but it's a minimal-effort part of your researching process. You want to make sure that the school's pass rate is above 90%. You might be thinking: what does the pass rate even mean? Why should I care? Although passing the Boards does require a lot of discipline and self-motivation, the better the teaching is at a school the more likely the students are to pass the Boards. Schools with a solid basic science curriculum and good review will put their applicants at an advantage when it comes to the Boards.

You may also want to find out the amount of time and flexibility schools allow for studying for Step 1 and Step 2, when they would need to be taken (important), and if they're required for graduation. Flexibility when taking the Steps is a key advantage that you should think about. Medical students typically take a month off to study for both exams, often studying every day, but your study habits may differ. For example, if you've been a procrastinator, you may value flexibility in extending your Boards study time. Flexibility also comes into play when you determine when schools require you to take the Boards. Some schools (like Tufts) compel you to take the Boards before you start clinics, others let you wait until you've had some clinical time (which puts the basic science curriculum into a practical context, making studying easier), while a few (like the University of Pennsylvania) don't set any parameters for when you take the Boards.

8.5.3   Residency Match

Almost every school includes a list of their recent graduating class' match list in your interview packet. Through this list, schools may brag about the top programs at which their applicants are matching and reassure applicants that most of their students match. Examine this match list to see how many students match in the specialties you are considering, and where they are matching. If you're not yet sure at all what you want to do, and are interested in keeping your options open, you should check out match rates in the more competitive specialties: anesthesia, dermatology, radiology, radiation oncology, ophthalmology, and plastic surgery. These will give you an indication of the school's overall competitiveness in the match process and a measure of how much each medical school invests in helping its students succeed in the process. Remember, not all medical students match, and many of these students end up in specialties in which they are not really interested. Match rates in general, are important, but particularly in competitive specialties.

8.5.4 Strengths in Your Areas of Interest

If you are really stuck choosing between schools, expand your investigations from Researching Schools III. Spend some additional time looking into each school's prominence, strengths, and offerings in areas related to your ambition and interests. If you are fortunate enough to go on a second-look, take some time to meet with faculty in the departments that interest you. Though they're probably busy, they'll usually take some time to meet with you or offer to communicate via email. If they're not happy to fuel your interest in their work, or are evasive, that's a big red flag; if they won't give you the time of day as a prospective student, what does that say about how you will be treated if you actually attend the school.

When you speak to faculty or students about your area of interest, you will want to explore existing opportunities for students to get involved in field activities or research, how (or if) students are selected, and what impact these experiences have had on students' career trajectory. For example, if several students showed initiative and recently co-authored a journal article on plastic surgery, this is a good sign that if you make an effort at this institution, there is a good chance it will pay off. However, if it appears that only students in Alpha Omega Alpha (medical schools' honor society; *very* difficult to be inducted) have any involvement on projects, or that students aren't involved at all, you shouldn't count on being a pioneer in establishing opportunities—medical school is hard enough!

8.5.5 Lifestyle

Lifestyle is probably one of the most important factors in choosing a medical school, yet it is often the one that is the most difficult to assess. When you go to second-look weekend, medical schools look more like a fun sequence of parties and group events. That makes medical school seem like a chilled-out world with a cohesive community. Don't let your capacity for critical thought take a vacation during this process. What do you ask, whom do you ask, and when?

This part is tricky. In researching lifestyle, there are a couple of things you should recognize. First of all, the students that communicate with prospective students may be self-selected; they are normally the students who really like their medical school. You may interact with a wider variety of students during lunch or mixers that lure in all types of students with free food. If you happen to converse with a seemingly cool student during your visit, don't be shy to get his or her email address; just tell them you'd appreciate being able to contact them in case you have any questions when it comes time to decide among schools. You don't want to go around asking every student you meet for their contact info. If you've just had a 5-10 minute conversation with one, however, such a request is natural. It is helpful to ask students what they would improve about their school, or what medical school they would select if they could choose again. Questions such as these will help you learn about some of the school's downsides and whether students seem happy there. In general, the more specific and simple your questions are, the easier your information gathering will be. For example, "About how many hours a day do you study?" is going to get a more realistic answer than asking, "What percentage of your time do you devote to studying?"

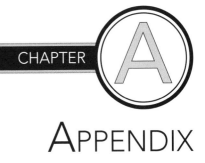

APPENDIX

A.1 OUR MED SCHOOL SLANG: GLOSSARY OF TERMINOLOGY

We throw around a fair amount of jargon in this book. Most of it is clear in context; however, if you are unfamiliar with these terms, here is the place to get clarification.

BCPM GPA/Designation—The GPA calculated from courses designated as BCPM, or biological sciences, chemistry, physics, and mathematics courses. AMCAS provides guidelines on which courses are BCPM (a chart is included in **Chapter 3**). The BCPM GPA is a very important determinant in an applicant's competitiveness, often moreso than overall GPA.

Cardinal Questions—Fundamental questions that you must ask yourself in order to clarify your goals and motivations in medicine, so that you may maximize your potential in the application and interview (See **Chapter 4** and **Chapter 6**).

Extracurriculars—short-hand for extracurricular activities, or any activity that is outside the curriculum of study and is pursued voluntarily.

Gift Wrap—Even when it's not Christmas, the **Gift Wrap** (explained in depth in **Chapter 4**) is the theme surrounding your personal statement that makes your essay memorable.

Five Golden Steps—No pyrite here. Our Five Golden Steps guide your way to go to construction of an effective personal statement (see **Chapter 4**).

MuD-PhuD—Endearing terms used to describe medical students in MD/PhD programs.

Six Platinum Steps—Not your average credit card. Really, it's our six-step approach to preparing and executing a polished, effective **Sales Pitch** and interview (see **Chapter 6**).

Postbac—This is not a post-operative spinal-surgery patient. It is short for post-baccalaureate, and the term encompasses organized programs that offer students already possessing a bachelor's degree science courses that fulfill pre-medical requirements.

Sales Pitch—Your story for the interview, which strategically emphasizes your answers to the three **Cardinal Questions**, allowing you to put your best foot forward during interviews (see **Chapter 6**).

Secondary—A supplemental application to the AMCAS primary application; indicates passage into Phase 2 of the application process. Some schools screen candidates before sending a secondary; many do not (see **Chapter 5**).

Second-look—A weekend or longer event, usually held between March and May, during which admitted students are invited to a more in-depth orientation to schools (see **Chapter 8**).

Self-Reflection Chart—A chart in which you can list your experiences and positive attributes as well as articulate your goals; this will assist you in writing an optimal personal statement (see **Chapter 4**).

A.2 APPLICATION TIMELINE: OVERVIEW

Planner's Timeline	"Vanilla on the Inside" (The In-betweeners)	Procastinator's Timeline
Spring Junior Year (or 18 months prior to planned matriculation)	**Spring Junior Year** (or 18 months prior to planned matriculation)	**Spring Junior Year** (or 18 months prior to planned matriculation)
• *Get your creative juices flowing by churning through the 5 Steps of the Personal Statement (Chapter 4). Have your topic solidified by the time you take the MCAT.*	• *Add the personal statement on your list of "things I need to do if I have extra time." Casually think about the topic over cocktails.*	• *18 months? That's like over 540 days. Don't freak out over something due next century.*
Early May	**Early May**	**Early May**
• ***AMCAS application becomes available online.*** *Become familiar with its format and requirements.* • ***Finish your draft.*** *Start shopping your statement around to your proofreaders, add finishing touches.*	• *AMCAS application available online—get a user ID and password before you forget.* • *Chat with your friends about getting some topics.* • *Take a glance at Chapter 4, The 5 Steps to Writing a Personal Statement.*	• *Dude, you just gotta make sure you apply on time for a test date before August.*
Early June	**Early June**	**Early June**
• ***Earliest AMCAS application can be submitted.*** *Finish the other sections, and make sure it's ready to go to avoid the rush. Most top schools have rolling admissions.*	• *AMCAS application can be turned in—why rush? Turn in something you're proud of. Now that summer's here, use your free time to solidify your topic choice and get a draft going.*	• *Miami is great this time of year.*
July	**July**	**July**
• ***Secondary applications sent.*** *If you've made initial cuts, you'll start receiving secondary applications. Return them within two weeks of receipt.*	• *Start filling in the other parts of your online AMCAS application.* • *Shop your draft around to proofreaders. You're still okay, but keep in mind admissions is rolling.*	• *Get your online user ID and password set up in that internet café by the beach on the Costa del Sol.*

September	Late August/September	September
• **First invitations for interviews sent.** Start scheduling dates by geographic location to minimize travel. • **Finalize your sales pitch!** (See chapter 6)	• *Finalize your proofreads and submit your AMCAS app—the earlier the better.* • *Return your secondaries within 2 ½ to 3 weeks of receipt.*	• *Whip out the 5 Steps and get cracking. Hopefully your summertime bliss will have you refreshed and inspired.* • *Shop your draft for proofreads within the week.* • ***Submit your primary AMCAS application by midnight October 15th***, *or your list of potential schools will dwindle quickly.* • ***Ensure that your transcripts arrive at AMCAS no later than 14 days after the school's deadline.*** *Don't skimp here. Registrars are complacent career bureaucrats—your urgency will ring hollow to them. After the 14 days, your application will be tossed out.*
October/November/December	**October/November**	**November/December**
• **Interviews!** *Take detailed notes about each school so you don't forget. Keep your pitch focused and don't let travel bog you down.*	• *Respond promptly to interview requests and start shopping for that suit!* • *Formulate your pitch (Chapter 6) and remember each school's feel and layout—after number six or seven, it's harder to remember who gave two more weeks of electives and who gave free parking.*	• *Secondaries should start to arrive—get them back ASAP.* • *Some schools have final deadlines in November and December— add to your list if need be.* • *Top schools will interview through mid-February—if you don't score that interview, call them up! Chances are they might have an opening on their last dates.*

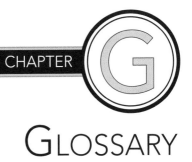

GLOSSARY

ALLOPATHIC SCHOOLS

ALBANY MEDICAL COLLEGE

47 New Scotland Avenue, Mail Code 3
Albany, NY 12208
Phone: 518-262-5521
Fax: 518-262-5887
admissions@mail.amc.edu
www.amc.edu

TOTAL ENROLLMENT: 538

% ACCEPTED: 4.60%

% MALE/FEMALE RATIO: 45/55

% UNDERREP. MINORITIES: 8%

APPLICATION DEADLINE: 11/15

APPLICATION NOTIFICATION: 12/1

EARLY APPLICATION DEADLINE: NA

EARLY APPLICATION NOTIFICATION: NA

TRANSFERS ACCEPTED: No

ADMISSIONS DEFFERABLE: Yes

APPLICATION FEE: $100

INTERVIEW TIMEFRAMES: Sept-April

MCAT SCORES: 29.4

GPA: 3.5

IN-STATE TUITION: $50,002

OUT-OF-STATE TUITION: $50,002

TYPE OF SCHOOL: Private

UNIVERSITY OF THE CARIBBEAN

School of Medicine
Medical Education Administrative Services
901 Ponce De Leon Blvd., Suite 401
Coral Gables, FL 33134
Phone: 866-372-2282
Fax: 786-433-0974
admissions@aucmed.edu
www.aucmed.edu

TOTAL ENROLLMENT: 828

% ACCEPTED: 47.00%

% MALE/FEMALE RATIO: 58/42

% UNDERREP. MINORITIES: NA

APPLICATION DEADLINE: Rolling

APPLICATION NOTIFICATION: Rolling

EARLY APPLICATION DEADLINE: NA

EARLY APPLICATION NOTIFICATION: NA

TRANSFERS ACCEPTED: Yes

ADMISSIONS DEFFERABLE: Yes

APPLICATION FEE: $75

INTERVIEW TIMEFRAMES: NA

MCAT SCORES: 22.6

GPA: 3.1

IN-STATE TUITION: $39,600

OUT-OF-STATE TUITION: $39,600

TYPE OF SCHOOL: Private/international Not Accredited

BAYLOR COLLEGE OF MEDICINE

Office of Admissions Information
1 Baylor Plaza
Houston, TX 77 030
Phone: 713-798-4842
Fax: 713-798-5563
admissions@bcm.edu
www.bcm.edu

TOTAL ENROLLMENT: 673

% ACCEPTED: 6.70%

% MALE/FEMALE RATIO: 52/48

% UNDERREP. MINORITIES: 19%

APPLICATION DEADLINE: 11/1

APPLICATION NOTIFICATION: Rolling

EARLY APPLICATION DEADLINE: 6/1

EARLY APPLICATION NOTIFICATION: 10/1

TRANSFERS ACCEPTED: Yes

ADMISSIONS DEFFERABLE: Yes

APPLICATION FEE: $70

INTERVIEW TIMEFRAMES: September-February

MCAT SCORES: NA

GPA: 3.8

IN-STATE TUITION: $44,511

OUT-OF-STATE TUITION: $44,511

TYPE OF SCHOOL: Private

BOSTON UNIVERSITY

715 Albany Street
Boston, MA 02118
Phone: 617-638-4630
Fax: 617-638-4718
medadms@bu.edu
www.bumc.bu.edu

TOTAL ENROLLMENT: 632

% ACCEPTED: 4.73%

% MALE/FEMALE RATIO: 47/53

% UNDERREP. MINORITIES: 16%

APPLICATION DEADLINE: 11/1

APPLICATION NOTIFICATION: Rolling

EARLY APPLICATION DEADLINE: 8/1

EARLY APPLICATION NOTIFICATION: 10/1

TRANSFERS ACCEPTED: No

ADMISSIONS DEFFERABLE: No

APPLICATION FEE: $100

INTERVIEW TIMEFRAMES: October-February

MCAT SCORES: 32.06

GPA: 3.65

IN-STATE TUITION: $53,494

OUT-OF-STATE TUITION: $53,494

TYPE OF SCHOOL: Private

BROWN UNIVERSITY

Brown Medical School
97 Waterman Street, Box G-A213
Providence, RI 02912
Phone: 401-863-2149
Fax: 401-863-3801
medschool_admissions@brown.edu

bms.brown.edu/med

TOTAL ENROLLMENT: 345

% ACCEPTED: 4.30%

% MALE/FEMALE RATIO: 42/58

% UNDERREP. MINORITIES: 44%

APPLICATION DEADLINE: 11/1

APPLICATION NOTIFICATION: Rolling

EARLY APPLICATION DEADLINE: NA

EARLY APPLICATION NOTIFICATION: NA

TRANSFERS ACCEPTED: Yes

ADMISSIONS DEFFERABLE: Yes

APPLICATION FEE: $85

INTERVIEW TIMEFRAMES: NA

MCAT SCORES: 33.4

GPA: 3.62

IN-STATE TUITION: $54,717

OUT-OF-STATE TUITION: $54,717

TYPE OF SCHOOL: Private

CASE WESTERN RESERVE UNIVERSITY

School of Medicine
Associate Dean of Admissions
10900 Euclid Avenue
Cleveland, OH 44106
Phone: 216-368-2000
Fax: 216-368-4621
axh65@case.edu

casemed.case.edu

TOTAL ENROLLMENT: 132

% ACCEPTED: 7.44%

% MALE/FEMALE RATIO: 50/50

% UNDERREP. MINORITIES: 46%

APPLICATION DEADLINE: NA

APPLICATION NOTIFICATION: NA

EARLY APPLICATION DEADLINE: 11/15

EARLY APPLICATION NOTIFICATION: 1/15

TRANSFERS ACCEPTED: Yes

ADMISSIONS DEFFERABLE: Yes

APPLICATION FEE: $60

INTERVIEW TIMEFRAMES: September-March

MCAT SCORES: NA

GPA: NA

IN-STATE TUITION: $45,734

OUT-OF-STATE TUITION: $45,734

TYPE OF SCHOOL: Private

COLUMBIA UNIVERSITY

College of Physicians and Surgeons
Admissions Office
630 West 168th Street
P.O. Box 41
New York, NY 10032
Phone: 212-305-3595
Fax: 212-305-3601
psadmissions@columbia.edu
cumc.columbia.edu/dept/ps

TOTAL ENROLLMENT: 149

% ACCEPTED: 7.20%

% MALE/FEMALE RATIO: NA

% UNDERREP. MINORITIES: 12%

APPLICATION DEADLINE: 11/15

APPLICATION NOTIFICATION: 3/1

EARLY APPLICATION DEADLINE: NA

EARLY APPLICATION NOTIFICATION: NA

TRANSFERS ACCEPTED: Yes

ADMISSIONS DEFFERABLE: Yes

APPLICATION FEE: $75

INTERVIEW TIMEFRAMES: September-March

MCAT SCORES: 35.4

GPA: 3.7

IN-STATE TUITION: $56,650

OUT-OF-STATE TUITION: $56,650

TYPE OF SCHOOL: Private

CORNELL UNIVERSITY

Joan & Sanford I. Weill Medical College
Office of Admissions
445 East 69th Street
New York, NY 10021
Phone: 212-746-1067
Fax: 212-746-8052
cumc-admissions@med.cornell.edu
www.med.cornell.edu

TOTAL ENROLLMENT: 412

% ACCEPTED: 5.06%

% MALE/FEMALE RATIO: 50/50

% UNDERREP. MINORITIES: NA

APPLICATION DEADLINE: 10/15

APPLICATION NOTIFICATION: 3/10

EARLY APPLICATION DEADLINE: 8/1

EARLY APPLICATION NOTIFICATION: 10/1

TRANSFERS ACCEPTED: Yes

ADMISSIONS DEFFERABLE: Yes

APPLICATION FEE: $75

INTERVIEW TIMEFRAMES: October-February

MCAT SCORES: 34.6

GPA: 3.72

IN-STATE TUITION: $45,422

OUT-OF-STATE TUITION: $45,422

TYPE OF SCHOOL: Private

CREIGHTON UNIVERSITY

School of Medicine
Office of Admissions
2500 California Plaza
Omaha, NE 68178
Phone: 402-280-2799
Fax: 402-280-1241
medschadm@creighton.edu
medicine.creighton.edu

TOTAL ENROLLMENT: 460

% ACCEPTED: 8.00%

% MALE/FEMALE RATIO: 54/48

% UNDERREP. MINORITIES: 8%

APPLICATION DEADLINE: 12/1

APPLICATION NOTIFICATION: Rolling

EARLY APPLICATION DEADLINE: 6/1-8/1

EARLY APPLICATION NOTIFICATION: 10/1

TRANSFERS ACCEPTED: Yes

ADMISSIONS DEFFERABLE: Yes

APPLICATION FEE: $75

INTERVIEW TIMEFRAMES: September-spring

MCAT SCORES: 29.4

GPA: 3.7

IN-STATE TUITION: $57,960

OUT-OF-STATE TUITION: $57,960

TYPE OF SCHOOL: Private

DALHOUSIE UNIVERSITY

Faculty of Medicine
5849 University Avenue
Halifax, Nova Scotia, Canada B3H 4H7
Phone: 902-494-1874
Fax: 902-494-6369
medicine.admissions@dal.ca
www.admissions.medicine.dal.ca

TOTAL ENROLLMENT: 91

% ACCEPTED: 15.70%

% MALE/FEMALE RATIO: 37/63

% UNDERREP. MINORITIES: 37%

APPLICATION DEADLINE: 10/31

APPLICATION NOTIFICATION: 3/1

EARLY APPLICATION DEADLINE: NA

EARLY APPLICATION NOTIFICATION: NA

TRANSFERS ACCEPTED: No

ADMISSIONS DEFFERABLE: No

APPLICATION FEE: $70

INTERVIEW TIMEFRAMES: NA

MCAT SCORES: 29

GPA: 3.5

IN-STATE TUITION: $15,480

OUT-OF-STATE TUITION: $21,120

TYPE OF SCHOOL: Public

DARTMOUTH COLLEGE

Dartmouth Medical School
3 Rope Ferry Road
Hanover, NH 03755-1404
Phone: 603-650-1505
Fax: 603-650-1560
dmsadmissions@dartmouth.edu

www.dms.dartmouth.edu

TOTAL ENROLLMENT: 298

% ACCEPTED: 5.71%

% MALE/FEMALE RATIO: 50/50

% UNDERREP. MINORITIES: NA

APPLICATION DEADLINE: 11/1

APPLICATION NOTIFICATION: Rolling

EARLY APPLICATION DEADLINE: NA

EARLY APPLICATION NOTIFICATION: NA

TRANSFERS ACCEPTED: Yes

ADMISSIONS DEFFERABLE: Yes

APPLICATION FEE: $75

INTERVIEW TIMEFRAMES: September-April

MCAT SCORES: 32.3

GPA: 3.7

IN-STATE TUITION: $46,525

OUT-OF-STATE TUITION: $46,525

TYPE OF SCHOOL: Private

DREXEL UNIVERSITY

College of Medicine
2900 Queen Lane
Philadelphia, PA 19129
Phone: 215-991-8202
Fax: 215-843-1766
medadms@drexel.edu

www.drexelmed.edu

TOTAL ENROLLMENT: 1016

% ACCEPTED: 13.07%

% MALE/FEMALE RATIO: 50/50

% UNDERREP. MINORITIES: 15%

APPLICATION DEADLINE: 12/1

APPLICATION NOTIFICATION: 10/15

EARLY APPLICATION DEADLINE: 8/1

EARLY APPLICATION NOTIFICATION: 10/5

TRANSFERS ACCEPTED: Yes

ADMISSIONS DEFFERABLE: Yes

APPLICATION FEE: $75

INTERVIEW TIMEFRAMES: September-April

MCAT SCORES: 31

GPA: 3.5

IN-STATE TUITION: $59,545

OUT-OF-STATE TUITION: $59,545

TYPE OF SCHOOL: Private

DUKE UNIVERSITY

School of Medicine
Committee on Admissions
P.O. Box 3710, DUMC
Durham, NC 27710
Phone: 919-684-2985
Fax: 919-684-8893
medadm@mc.duke.edu

medschool.duke.edu

TOTAL ENROLLMENT: 402

% ACCEPTED: 3.64%

% MALE/FEMALE RATIO: 53/47

% UNDERREP. MINORITIES: 18%

APPLICATION DEADLINE: 11/1

APPLICATION NOTIFICATION: 3/1

EARLY APPLICATION DEADLINE: NA

EARLY APPLICATION NOTIFICATION: NA

TRANSFERS ACCEPTED: No

ADMISSIONS DEFFERABLE: Yes

APPLICATION FEE: $80

INTERVIEW TIMEFRAMES: September-February

MCAT SCORES: 33

GPA: 3.8

IN-STATE TUITION: $57,320

OUT-OF-STATE TUITION: $57,320

TYPE OF SCHOOL: Private

EAST CAROLINA UNIVERSITY

Brody School of Medicine
Office of Admissions
600 Moye Boulevard
Greenville, NC 27834
Phone: 252-744-2202
Fax: 252-744-1926
somadmissions@mail.edu.edu

www.ecu.edu/bsomadmissions

TOTAL ENROLLMENT: 288

% ACCEPTED: 8.30%

% MALE/FEMALE RATIO: 50/50

% UNDERREP. MINORITIES: 34%

APPLICATION DEADLINE: 11/15

APPLICATION NOTIFICATION: Rolling

EARLY APPLICATION DEADLINE: 6/1-8/1

EARLY APPLICATION NOTIFICATION: 10/1

TRANSFERS ACCEPTED: Yes

ADMISSIONS DEFFERABLE: No

APPLICATION FEE: $60

INTERVIEW TIMEFRAMES: August-April

MCAT SCORES: 27

GPA: 3.5

IN-STATE TUITION: $8,831

OUT-OF-STATE TUITION: $33,521

TYPE OF SCHOOL: Public

EAST TENNESSEE STATE UNIVERSITY

James H. Quillen College of Medicine
P.O. Box 70580
Johnson City, TN 37614-1708
Phone: 423-439-2033
Fax: 423-439-2110
sacom@etsu.edu

com.etst.edu

TOTAL ENROLLMENT: NA

% ACCEPTED: NA

% MALE/FEMALE RATIO: NA

% UNDERREP. MINORITIES: NA

APPLICATION DEADLINE: 11/15

APPLICATION NOTIFICATION: 7/1

EARLY APPLICATION DEADLINE: 6/1-8/1

EARLY APPLICATION NOTIFICATION: 10/1

TRANSFERS ACCEPTED: Yes

ADMISSIONS DEFFERABLE: Yes

APPLICATION FEE: $50

INTERVIEW TIMEFRAMES: September-March

MCAT SCORES: NA

GPA: NA

IN-STATE TUITION: $28,303

OUT-OF-STATE TUITION: $43,245

TYPE OF SCHOOL: Public

EASTERN VIRGINIA SCHOOL

Office of Admissions
700 West Olney Road
Norfolk, VA 23507-1607
Phone: 757-446-5812
Fax: 757-446-5896
nanezkf@evms.edu

www.evms.edu

TOTAL ENROLLMENT: 432

% ACCEPTED: 13.10%

% MALE/FEMALE RATIO: 47/53

% UNDERREP. MINORITIES: 12%

APPLICATION DEADLINE: 11/15

APPLICATION NOTIFICATION: Rolling

EARLY APPLICATION DEADLINE: 6/1-8/1

EARLY APPLICATION NOTIFICATION: 10/1

TRANSFERS ACCEPTED: Yes

ADMISSIONS DEFFERABLE: Yes

APPLICATION FEE: $90

INTERVIEW TIMEFRAMES: September-March

MCAT SCORES: 29.3

GPA: 3.5

IN-STATE TUITION: $22,941

OUT-OF-STATE TUITION: $22,941

TYPE OF SCHOOL: Private

Emory University

School of Medicine
1440 Clifton Road NE, Suite 115
Atlanta, GA 30322-4510
Phone: 404-727-5660
Fax: 404-727-5456
medadmiss@emory.edu
www.med.emory.edu

Total Enrollment: 462

% Accepted: 8.20%

% Male/Female Ratio: 51/49

% Underrep. Minorities: 28%

Application Deadline: 10/15

Application Notification: Rollinig

Early Application Deadline: NA

Early Application Notification: NA

Transfers Accepted: Yes

Admissions Defferable: Yes

Application Fee: $80

Interview Timeframes: October-February

MCAT Scores: 33.3

GPA: 3.64

In-state Tuition: $56,210

Out-of-state Tuition: $56,210

Type of School: Private

Florida State University

College of Medicine
Admissions Office
1115 West Call Street
Tallahassee, FL 32306-4300
Phone: 850-644-7904
Fax: 850-645-1420
medinformation@med.fsu.edu
www.med.fsy.edu/

Total Enrollment: 115

% Accepted: 21.00%

% Male/Female Ratio: 61/39

% Underrep. Minorities: 31%

Application Deadline: 12/1

Application Notification: 4/15

Early Application Deadline: 8/1

Early Application Notification: 9/3

Transfers Accepted: No

Admissions Defferable: Yes

Application Fee: NA

Interview Timeframes: September-March

MCAT Scores: 26.6

GPA: 3.6

In-state Tuition: $28,624

Out-of-state Tuition: NA

Type of School: Public

THE GEORGE WASHINGTON UNIVERSITY

School of Medicine and Health Sciences
Office of Admissions
2300 I Street, NW
Ross Hall 716
Washington, DC 20037
Phone: 202-994-3506
Fax: 202-994-1753
medadmit@gwu.edu
www.gwumc.edu/edu/admis

TOTAL ENROLLMENT: 675

% ACCEPTED: 4.60%

% MALE/FEMALE RATIO: 45/55

% UNDERREP. MINORITIES: 16%

APPLICATION DEADLINE: 12/1

APPLICATION NOTIFICATION: Rolling

EARLY APPLICATION DEADLINE: 6/1-8/1

EARLY APPLICATION NOTIFICATION: 10/1

TRANSFERS ACCEPTED: Yes

ADMISSIONS DEFFERABLE: Yes

APPLICATION FEE: $105

INTERVIEW TIMEFRAMES: September-March

MCAT SCORES: 28.75

GPA: 3.55

IN-STATE TUITION: $60,470

OUT-OF-STATE TUITION: $60,470

TYPE OF SCHOOL: Private

GEORGETOWN UNIVERSITY

School of Medicine
Office of Admissions
3900 Reservoir Road, NW
Washington, DC 20007
Phone: 202-687-1154
medicaladmissions@georgetown.edu
som.georgetown.edu/

TOTAL ENROLLMENT: 699

% ACCEPTED: NA

% MALE/FEMALE RATIO: 56/44

% UNDERREP. MINORITIES: 26%

APPLICATION DEADLINE: 10/20

APPLICATION NOTIFICATION: 10/15

EARLY APPLICATION DEADLINE: NA

EARLY APPLICATION NOTIFICATION: NA

TRANSFERS ACCEPTED: Yes

ADMISSIONS DEFFERABLE: NA

APPLICATION FEE: $130

INTERVIEW TIMEFRAMES: September-May

MCAT SCORES: NA

GPA: 3.6

IN-STATE TUITION: $47,319

OUT-OF-STATE TUITION: $47,319

TYPE OF SCHOOL: Private

HARVARD UNIVERSITY

Harvard Medical School
Office of Admissions
210 Gordon Hall
25 Shattuck Street
Boston, MA 02115
Phone: 617-432-1550
Fax: 617-432-3307
admissions_Office@hms.harvard.edu
www.hms.harvard.edu

TOTAL ENROLLMENT: 735

% ACCEPTED: 4.63%

% MALE/FEMALE RATIO: 43/57

% UNDERREP. MINORITIES: 22%

APPLICATION DEADLINE: 10/15

APPLICATION NOTIFICATION: 3/7

EARLY APPLICATION DEADLINE: NA

EARLY APPLICATION NOTIFICATION: NA

TRANSFERS ACCEPTED: No

ADMISSIONS DEFFERABLE: Yes

APPLICATION FEE: $85

INTERVIEW TIMEFRAMES: September-January

MCAT SCORES: 35.05

GPA: 3.79

IN-STATE TUITION: $62,545

OUT-OF-STATE TUITION: $62,545

TYPE OF SCHOOL: Private

HOWARD UNIVERSITY

College of Medicine
Admissions Office
520 West Street, NW
Washington, DC 20059
Phone: 202-806-6270
Fax: 202-806-7934
shumphrey@howard.edu
www.med.howard.edu

TOTAL ENROLLMENT: 454

% ACCEPTED: 7.50%

% MALE/FEMALE RATIO: 51/49

% UNDERREP. MINORITIES: 59%

APPLICATION DEADLINE: 12/15

APPLICATION NOTIFICATION: 10/15

EARLY APPLICATION DEADLINE: NA

EARLY APPLICATION NOTIFICATION: NA

TRANSFERS ACCEPTED: No

ADMISSIONS DEFFERABLE: Yes

APPLICATION FEE: $45

INTERVIEW TIMEFRAMES: NA

MCAT SCORES: NA

GPA: NA

IN-STATE TUITION: $16,883

OUT-OF-STATE TUITION: $16,883

TYPE OF SCHOOL: Private

INDIANA UNIVERSITY

School of Medicine
Admissions Office
1120 South Drive
Fesler Hall 213
Indianapolis, IN 46202
Phone: 317-274-3772
Fax: 317-278-0211
inmedadm@iupui.edu
www.medicine.iu.edu/

TOTAL ENROLLMENT: 1159

% ACCEPTED: 14.82%

% MALE/FEMALE RATIO: 55/45

% UNDERREP. MINORITIES: 11%

APPLICATION DEADLINE: 12/15

APPLICATION NOTIFICATION: 10/15

EARLY APPLICATION DEADLINE: 6/1-8/1

EARLY APPLICATION NOTIFICATION: 10/1

TRANSFERS ACCEPTED: Yes

ADMISSIONS DEFFERABLE: Yes

APPLICATION FEE: $50

INTERVIEW TIMEFRAMES: September-February

MCAT SCORES: 30

GPA: 3.68

IN-STATE TUITION: $36,415

OUT-OF-STATE TUITION: $55,269

TYPE OF SCHOOL: Private

JOHNS HOPKINS UNIVERSITY

School of Medicine
733 North Broadway, Suite G-49
Baltimore, MD 21205
Phone: 410-955-3182
Fax: 410-955-7494
somadmiss@jhmi.edu
www.hopkinsmedicine.org

TOTAL ENROLLMENT: 464

% ACCEPTED: 6.00%

% MALE/FEMALE RATIO: 55/45

% UNDERREP. MINORITIES: 14%

APPLICATION DEADLINE: 10/15

APPLICATION NOTIFICATION: Rolling

EARLY APPLICATION DEADLINE: 7/1-8/15

EARLY APPLICATION NOTIFICATION: 10/1

TRANSFERS ACCEPTED: No

ADMISSIONS DEFFERABLE: Yes

APPLICATION FEE: $75

INTERVIEW TIMEFRAMES: September-March

MCAT SCORES: 34.48

GPA: 3.84

IN-STATE TUITION: $46,935

OUT-OF-STATE TUITION: $46,935

TYPE OF SCHOOL: Private

LOMA LINDA UNIVERSITY

School of Medicine
Loma Linda, CA 92350
Phone: 909-558-1100
Fax: 909-824-4146
admissions.sm.app@llu.edu
www.llu.edu/llu/medicine

TOTAL ENROLLMENT: 661

% ACCEPTED: NA

% MALE/FEMALE RATIO: 59/41

% UNDERREP. MINORITIES: 6%

APPLICATION DEADLINE: 11/1

APPLICATION NOTIFICATION: 12/15

EARLY APPLICATION DEADLINE: 6/1-8/1

EARLY APPLICATION NOTIFICATION: 10/1

TRANSFERS ACCEPTED: No

ADMISSIONS DEFFERABLE: Yes

APPLICATION FEE: $55

INTERVIEW TIMEFRAMES: November-March

MCAT SCORES: NA

GPA: NA

IN-STATE TUITION: $24,949

OUT-OF-STATE TUITION: $24,949

TYPE OF SCHOOL: Private

LOUISIANA STATE UNIVERSITY

School of Medicine In New Orleans
Office of Admissions
1901 Perdido Street
P.O. Box P3-4
New Orleans, LA 70112
Phone: 504-568-6262
Fax: 504-568-7701
ms-admissions@lsuhsc.edu
www.medschool.lsuhsc.edu/admissions

TOTAL ENROLLMENT: 712

% ACCEPTED: NA

% MALE/FEMALE RATIO: 50/50

% UNDERREP. MINORITIES: 15%

APPLICATION DEADLINE: 11/15

APPLICATION NOTIFICATION: Rolling

EARLY APPLICATION DEADLINE: 9/1

EARLY APPLICATION NOTIFICATION: 10/1

TRANSFERS ACCEPTED: Yes

ADMISSIONS DEFFERABLE: Yes

APPLICATION FEE: $50

INTERVIEW TIMEFRAMES: October-April

MCAT SCORES: 27.5

GPA: 3.7

IN-STATE TUITION: NA

OUT-OF-STATE TUITION: NA

TYPE OF SCHOOL: Public

LOUISIANA STATE UNIVERSITY

School of Medicine In Shreveport
Admissions Office
150 Kings Highway
P.O. Box 33932
Shreveport, LA 71130-3932
Phone: 318-675-5190
Fax: 308-675-5244
shvadm@lsuhc.edu
www.lsuhc.edu

TOTAL ENROLLMENT: 391

% ACCEPTED: 2.60%

% MALE/FEMALE RATIO: 67/33

% UNDERREP. MINORITIES: 5%

APPLICATION DEADLINE: 11/15

APPLICATION NOTIFICATION: 10/15

EARLY APPLICATION DEADLINE: 6/1-8/1

EARLY APPLICATION NOTIFICATION: 10/1

TRANSFERS ACCEPTED: Yes

ADMISSIONS DEFFERABLE: Yes

APPLICATION FEE: $50

INTERVIEW TIMEFRAMES: September-March

MCAT SCORES: NA

GPA: NA

IN-STATE TUITION: NA

OUT-OF-STATE TUITION: $14,726

TYPE OF SCHOOL: Public

LOYOLA UNIVERSITY CHICAGO

Stritch School of Medicine
2160 South First Avenue
Maywood, IL 60153
Phone: 708-216-3229
www.meddean.lumc.edu

TOTAL ENROLLMENT: 544

% ACCEPTED: 6.60%

% MALE/FEMALE RATIO: 51/49

% UNDERREP. MINORITIES: 18%

APPLICATION DEADLINE: 11/15

APPLICATION NOTIFICATION: 10/15

EARLY APPLICATION DEADLINE: NA

EARLY APPLICATION NOTIFICATION: NA

TRANSFERS ACCEPTED: Yes

ADMISSIONS DEFFERABLE: Yes

APPLICATION FEE: $70

INTERVIEW TIMEFRAMES: September-April

MCAT SCORES: 29.6

GPA: 3.62

IN-STATE TUITION: $52,870

OUT-OF-STATE TUITION: $52,870

TYPE OF SCHOOL: Private

MARSHALL UNIVERSITY

Joan C. Edwards School of Medicine
Office of Admissions
1600 Medical Center Drive
Huntington, WV 25701
Phone: 800-544-8514
Fax: 304-691-1744
warren@marshall.edu
www.musom.marshall.edu

TOTAL ENROLLMENT: 211

% ACCEPTED: 13.00%

% MALE/FEMALE RATIO: 60/40

% UNDERREP. MINORITIES: 18%

APPLICATION DEADLINE: 12/1

APPLICATION NOTIFICATION: 10/15

EARLY APPLICATION DEADLINE: NA

EARLY APPLICATION NOTIFICATION: NA

TRANSFERS ACCEPTED: Yes

ADMISSIONS DEFFERABLE: Yes

APPLICATION FEE: $50

INTERVIEW TIMEFRAMES: September-February

MCAT SCORES: 26.2

GPA: 3.5

IN-STATE TUITION: $32,208

OUT-OF-STATE TUITION: $55,598

TYPE OF SCHOOL: Public

MAYO CLINIC COLLEGE OF MEDICINE

Mayo Medical School
200 First Street, SW
Rochester, MN 55905
Phone: 507-284-3671
Fax: 507-284-2634
medschooladmissions@Mayo.edu
www.Mayo.edu/mms

TOTAL ENROLLMENT: 166

% ACCEPTED: 2.40%

% MALE/FEMALE RATIO: 51/49

% UNDERREP. MINORITIES: 13%

APPLICATION DEADLINE: 11/1

APPLICATION NOTIFICATION: Rolling

EARLY APPLICATION DEADLINE: 8/1

EARLY APPLICATION NOTIFICATION: 10/1

TRANSFERS ACCEPTED: No

ADMISSIONS DEFFERABLE: Yes

APPLICATION FEE: $75

INTERVIEW TIMEFRAMES: September-March

MCAT SCORES: 32.8

GPA: 3.84

IN-STATE TUITION: $39,948

OUT-OF-STATE TUITION: $39,948

TYPE OF SCHOOL: Private

McGILL UNIVERSITY

Faculty of Medicine
3655 Sir William Osler Promenade
Suite 602
Montreal, QC H3G 1Y6
Phone: 1 514-398-3517
Fax: 1 514-398-4631
admissions.med@mcgill.ca

www.medicine.mcgill.ca/admissions

TOTAL ENROLLMENT: 731

% ACCEPTED: 2.42%

% MALE/FEMALE RATIO: 45/55

% UNDERREP. MINORITIES: NA

APPLICATION DEADLINE: 11/15

APPLICATION NOTIFICATION: 3/31

EARLY APPLICATION DEADLINE: NA

EARLY APPLICATION NOTIFICATION: 1/15

TRANSFERS ACCEPTED: No

ADMISSIONS DEFFERABLE: Yes

APPLICATION FEE: $80

INTERVIEW TIMEFRAMES: NA

MCAT SCORES: 32

GPA: 3.74

IN-STATE TUITION: $6,883

OUT-OF-STATE TUITION: $26,463

TYPE OF SCHOOL: Public

McMASTER UNIVERSITY

Undergraduate Medical Programme
1200 Main Street, Room: 1M7
Hamilton, ON L8N 3Z5
Phone: 905-525-9140
Fax: 905-546-0349
mdadmit@mcmaster.ca

www.fhs.mcmaster.ca/mdprog

TOTAL ENROLLMENT: NA

% ACCEPTED: 5.20%

% MALE/FEMALE RATIO: NA

% UNDERREP. MINORITIES: NA

APPLICATION DEADLINE: 10/1

APPLICATION NOTIFICATION: 5/31

EARLY APPLICATION DEADLINE: NA

EARLY APPLICATION NOTIFICATION: NA

TRANSFERS ACCEPTED: No

ADMISSIONS DEFFERABLE: Yes

APPLICATION FEE: NA

INTERVIEW TIMEFRAMES: March-April

MCAT SCORES: NA

GPA: 3.8

IN-STATE TUITION: $4,422

OUT-OF-STATE TUITION: NA

TYPE OF SCHOOL: Public

MEDICAL COLLEGE OF GEORGIA

School of Medicine
Office of Admissions, AA-2040
Augusta, GA 30912
Phone: 706-721-3186
Fax: 706-721-0959
sci.med.stdadmin@mail.mcg.edu

www.mcg.edu

TOTAL ENROLLMENT: 720

% ACCEPTED: 14.81%

% MALE/FEMALE RATIO: NA

% UNDERREP. MINORITIES: NA

APPLICATION DEADLINE: 11/1

APPLICATION NOTIFICATION: 5/1

EARLY APPLICATION DEADLINE: 6/1-8/1

EARLY APPLICATION NOTIFICATION: 10/1

TRANSFERS ACCEPTED: Yes

ADMISSIONS DEFFERABLE: Yes

APPLICATION FEE: NA

INTERVIEW TIMEFRAMES: October-March

MCAT SCORES: 30.19

GPA: 3.66

IN-STATE TUITION: $12,676

OUT-OF-STATE TUITION: $31,802

TYPE OF SCHOOL: Public

MEDICAL UNIVERSITY OF OHIO

College of Medicine
3045 Arlington Avenue
Toledo, OH 43614
Phone: 419-381-4229
Fax: 419-381-4005
admissions@meduohio.edu

www.meduohio.edu

TOTAL ENROLLMENT: 565

% ACCEPTED: 1.00%

% MALE/FEMALE RATIO: 70/30

% UNDERREP. MINORITIES: 10%

APPLICATION DEADLINE: 11/1

APPLICATION NOTIFICATION: 10/15

EARLY APPLICATION DEADLINE: 6/1-8/1

EARLY APPLICATION NOTIFICATION: 10/1

TRANSFERS ACCEPTED: Yes

ADMISSIONS DEFFERABLE: Yes

APPLICATION FEE: $30

INTERVIEW TIMEFRAMES: October-April

MCAT SCORES: NA

GPA: NA

IN-STATE TUITION: $13,307

OUT-OF-STATE TUITION: $25,761

TYPE OF SCHOOL: Public

MEDICAL COLLEGE OF WISCONSIN

Office of Admissions
8701 Watertown Plank Road
Milwaukee, WI 53226
Phone: 414-456-8246
Fax: 414-456-6505
www.medschool@mcw.edu
www.mcw.edu

TOTAL ENROLLMENT: 811

% ACCEPTED: 8.41%

% MALE/FEMALE RATIO: 56/44

% UNDERREP. MINORITIES: 10%

APPLICATION DEADLINE: 11/1

APPLICATION NOTIFICATION: 10/15

EARLY APPLICATION DEADLINE: 6/1-8/1

EARLY APPLICATION NOTIFICATION: 10/1

TRANSFERS ACCEPTED: Yes

ADMISSIONS DEFFERABLE: Yes

APPLICATION FEE: $60

INTERVIEW TIMEFRAMES: NA

MCAT SCORES: 29.7

GPA: 3.72

IN-STATE TUITION: $42,437

OUT-OF-STATE TUITION: $42,437

TYPE OF SCHOOL: Private

MEDICAL UNIVERSITY OF SOUTH CAROLINA

College of Medicine
96 Jonathan Lucas Street, Suite 601
P.O. Box 250617
Charleston, SC 29425
Phone: 843-792-2055
Fax: 843-792-4262
taylorwl@musc.edu
www2.musc.edu./com/com/html

TOTAL ENROLLMENT: 584

% ACCEPTED: 10.30%

% MALE/FEMALE RATIO: 55/45

% UNDERREP. MINORITIES: 14%

APPLICATION DEADLINE: 12/1

APPLICATION NOTIFICATION: Rolling

EARLY APPLICATION DEADLINE: 6/1-8/1

EARLY APPLICATION NOTIFICATION: 10/1

TRANSFERS ACCEPTED: Yes

ADMISSIONS DEFFERABLE: Yes

APPLICATION FEE: $55

INTERVIEW TIMEFRAMES: September-March

MCAT SCORES: 29

GPA: 3.6

IN-STATE TUITION: $27,022

OUT-OF-STATE TUITION: $51,342

TYPE OF SCHOOL: Public

MEHARRY MEDICAL COLLEGE

School of Medicine
1005 Dr. D.B. Todd Jr. Boulevard
Nashville, TN 37208-3599
Phone: 615-327-6223
Fax: 615-327-6228
admissions@mmc.edu
www.mmc.edu

TOTAL ENROLLMENT: 343

% ACCEPTED: 4.10%

% MALE/FEMALE RATIO: 48/52

% UNDERREP. MINORITIES: 48%

APPLICATION DEADLINE: 12/1

APPLICATION NOTIFICATION: 10/15

EARLY APPLICATION DEADLINE: 6/1-8/1

EARLY APPLICATION NOTIFICATION: 10/1

TRANSFERS ACCEPTED: No

ADMISSIONS DEFFERABLE: No

APPLICATION FEE: $60

INTERVIEW TIMEFRAMES: September-May

MCAT SCORES: NA

GPA: NA

IN-STATE TUITION: $28,652

OUT-OF-STATE TUITION: $28,652

TYPE OF SCHOOL: Private

MEMORIAL UNIVERSITY NEWFOUNDLAND

Faculty of Medicine
Room 1751, Health Sciences Center
St. John's, NFA1B 3V6
Phone: 709-777-6615
Fax: 709-777-8422
munmed@mun.ca
www.med.mun.ca/admissions

TOTAL ENROLLMENT: 244

% ACCEPTED: 11.90%

% MALE/FEMALE RATIO: 48/52

% UNDERREP. MINORITIES: NA

APPLICATION DEADLINE: 11/15

APPLICATION NOTIFICATION: 3/1

EARLY APPLICATION DEADLINE: NA

EARLY APPLICATION NOTIFICATION: NA

TRANSFERS ACCEPTED: No

ADMISSIONS DEFFERABLE: Yes

APPLICATION FEE: $75

INTERVIEW TIMEFRAMES: NA

MCAT SCORES: 27

GPA: 3.7

IN-STATE TUITION: $17,300

OUT-OF-STATE TUITION: $41,238

TYPE OF SCHOOL: Public

MERCER UNIVERSITY

School of Medicine
1550 College Street
Macon, GA 31207
Phone: 478-301-2542
Fax: 478-301-2547
faust_ek@mercer.edu
medicine.mercer.edu

TOTAL ENROLLMENT: 221

% ACCEPTED: 8.13%

% MALE/FEMALE RATIO: 58/42

% UNDERREP. MINORITIES: NA

APPLICATION DEADLINE: 11/1

APPLICATION NOTIFICATION: Rolling

EARLY APPLICATION DEADLINE: 6/1-8/1

EARLY APPLICATION NOTIFICATION: 10/1

TRANSFERS ACCEPTED: Yes

ADMISSIONS DEFFERABLE: Yes

APPLICATION FEE: $50

INTERVIEW TIMEFRAMES: October-March

MCAT SCORES: 25.33

GPA: 3.4

IN-STATE TUITION: $41,042

OUT-OF-STATE TUITION: $41,042

TYPE OF SCHOOL: Private

MICHIGAN STATE UNIVERSITY

College of Human Medicine
A-239 Life Sciences East
Lansing, MI 48824
Phone: 517-353-9620
Fax: 517-432-0021
mdadmissions@msu.edu
mdadmissions.msu.edu

TOTAL ENROLLMENT: 454

% ACCEPTED: 5.70%

% MALE/FEMALE RATIO: 43/57

% UNDERREP. MINORITIES: 36%

APPLICATION DEADLINE: 11/15

APPLICATION NOTIFICATION: Rolling

EARLY APPLICATION DEADLINE: 8/1

EARLY APPLICATION NOTIFICATION: 10/1

TRANSFERS ACCEPTED: Yes

ADMISSIONS DEFFERABLE: Yes

APPLICATION FEE: $60

INTERVIEW TIMEFRAMES: September-March

MCAT SCORES: 28.2

GPA: 3.52

IN-STATE TUITION: $38,924

OUT-OF-STATE TUITION: $66,824

TYPE OF SCHOOL: Public

MOREHOUSE COLLEGE

School of Medicine
Admissions and Student Affairs
720 Westview Drive, SW
atlanta, GA 30310
Phone: 404-752-1650
Fax: 404-752-1512
sroaf@msm.edu

www.msm.edu

TOTAL ENROLLMENT: 182

% ACCEPTED: 5.67%

% MALE/FEMALE RATIO: 37/63

% UNDERREP. MINORITIES: 87%

APPLICATION DEADLINE: 12/1

APPLICATION NOTIFICATION: 11/1

EARLY APPLICATION DEADLINE: 6/1-8/1

EARLY APPLICATION NOTIFICATION: 10/1

TRANSFERS ACCEPTED: Yes

ADMISSIONS DEFERRABLE: Yes

APPLICATION FEE: $50

INTERVIEW TIMEFRAMES: October-March

MCAT SCORES: NA

GPA: NA

IN-STATE TUITION: $45,120

OUT-OF-STATE TUITION: $45,120

TYPE OF SCHOOL: Private

NEW YORK MEDICAL COLLEGE

School of Medicine
Office of Admissions
Administration Building
Valhalla, NY 10595
Phone: 914-594-4507
Fax: 917-594-4976
mdadmit@nymc.edu

www.nymc.edu

TOTAL ENROLLMENT: 765

% ACCEPTED: 10.50%

% MALE/FEMALE RATIO: 50/50

% UNDERREP. MINORITIES: 10%

APPLICATION DEADLINE: 12/15

APPLICATION NOTIFICATION: Rolling

EARLY APPLICATION DEADLINE: 8/1

EARLY APPLICATION NOTIFICATION: 10/1

TRANSFERS ACCEPTED: Yes

ADMISSIONS DEFFERABLE: Yes

APPLICATION FEE: $100

INTERVIEW TIMEFRAMES: October-April

MCAT SCORES: 30.2

GPA: 3.5

IN-STATE TUITION: $59,252

OUT-OF-STATE TUITION: $59,252

TYPE OF SCHOOL: Private

NEW YORK UNIVERSITY

Mount Sinai School of Medicine
Annenberg 5-04A
P.O. Box 1002
1 Gustave L. Levy Place
New York, NY 10029-6574
Phone: 212-241-6696
Fax: 212-828-4135
admissions@mssm.edu
www.mssm.edu/bulletin

TOTAL ENROLLMENT: 473

% ACCEPTED: 7.70%

% MALE/FEMALE RATIO: 48/52

% UNDERREP. MINORITIES: 35%

APPLICATION DEADLINE: 11/1

APPLICATION NOTIFICATION: Rolling

EARLY APPLICATION DEADLINE: 8/1

EARLY APPLICATION NOTIFICATION: 10/1

TRANSFERS ACCEPTED: Yes

ADMISSIONS DEFFERABLE: Yes

APPLICATION FEE: $10

INTERVIEW TIMEFRAMES: September-March

MCAT SCORES: 33

GPA: 3.67

IN-STATE TUITION: $52,070

OUT-OF-STATE TUITION: $52,070

TYPE OF SCHOOL: Private

NEW YORK UNIVERSITY

School of Medicine
550 First Avenue
New York, NY 10016
Phone: 212-263-5290
Fax: 212-263-0720
admissions@med.nyu.edu
www.med.nyu.edu

TOTAL ENROLLMENT: 102

% ACCEPTED: 5.83%

% MALE/FEMALE RATIO: 51/49

% UNDERREP. MINORITIES: 9%

APPLICATION DEADLINE: 10/15

APPLICATION NOTIFICATION: 2/15

EARLY APPLICATION DEADLINE: NA

EARLY APPLICATION NOTIFICATION: NA

TRANSFERS ACCEPTED: No

ADMISSIONS DEFFERABLE: Yes

APPLICATION FEE: $100

INTERVIEW TIMEFRAMES: September-December

MCAT SCORES: 32.8

GPA: 3.73

IN-STATE TUITION: $53,125

OUT-OF-STATE TUITION: $53,125

TYPE OF SCHOOL: Private

NORTHEASTERN OHIO UNIVERSITIES

College of Medicine
P.O. Box 95
Rootstown, OH 44272-0095
Phone: 330-325-6270
Fax: 330-325-8372
admission@neoucom.edu
www.neoucom.edu

TOTAL ENROLLMENT: 430

% ACCEPTED: 18.12%

% MALE/FEMALE RATIO: 46/54

% UNDERREP. MINORITIES: 6%

APPLICATION DEADLINE: 11/1

APPLICATION NOTIFICATION: 3/21

EARLY APPLICATION DEADLINE: 6/1-8/1

EARLY APPLICATION NOTIFICATION: 10/1

TRANSFERS ACCEPTED: Yes

ADMISSIONS DEFFERABLE: No

APPLICATION FEE: $30

INTERVIEW TIMEFRAMES: November-March

MCAT SCORES: 27.4

GPA: 3.66

IN-STATE TUITION: $37,699

OUT-OF-STATE TUITION: $58,144

TYPE OF SCHOOL: Public

NORTHWESTERN UNIVERSITY

Feinberg School of Medicine
Admissions Office, 1st FLoor, Room 606
303 East Chicago Avenue
Chicago, IL 60611-3008
Phone: 312-503-8206
Fax: 312-503-0550
med-admissions@northwestern.edu
med-admissions.northwestern.edu

TOTAL ENROLLMENT: 678

% ACCEPTED: 5.60%

% MALE/FEMALE RATIO: 51/49

% UNDERREP. MINORITIES: 12%

APPLICATION DEADLINE: 10/15

APPLICATION NOTIFICATION: 12/15

EARLY APPLICATION DEADLINE: NA

EARLY APPLICATION NOTIFICATION: NA

TRANSFERS ACCEPTED: Yes

ADMISSIONS DEFFERABLE: Yes

APPLICATION FEE: $75

INTERVIEW TIMEFRAMES: October-February

MCAT SCORES: 33.8

GPA: 3.72

IN-STATE TUITION: $57,203

OUT-OF-STATE TUITION: $57,203

TYPE OF SCHOOL: Private

THE OHIO STATE UNIVERSITY

College of Medicine
155 D. Meiling Hall
370 West 9th Avenue
Columbus, OH 43210
Phone: 614-292-7137
Fax: 614-247-7959
medicine@osu.edu
www.medicine.osu.edu

TOTAL ENROLLMENT: 839

% ACCEPTED: 9.60%

% MALE/FEMALE RATIO: 63/37

% UNDERREP. MINORITIES: 32%

APPLICATION DEADLINE: 12/1

APPLICATION NOTIFICATION: 10/15

EARLY APPLICATION DEADLINE: 8/1

EARLY APPLICATION NOTIFICATION: 10/1

TRANSFERS ACCEPTED: Yes

ADMISSIONS DEFFERABLE: Yes

APPLICATION FEE: $60

INTERVIEW TIMEFRAMES: September-March

MCAT SCORES: 32.48

GPA: 3.72

IN-STATE TUITION: $41,100

OUT-OF-STATE TUITION: $53,911

TYPE OF SCHOOL: Public

OREGON HEALTH AND SCIENCE UNIVERSITY

School of Medicine
Office of Education & Student Affairs, L102
3181 Southwest
Portland, OR 97201
Phone: 503-494-2998
Fax: 503-494-3400
mdadmiss@ohsu.edu
www.ohsu.edu/edu/som-dean/admit.html

TOTAL ENROLLMENT: 452

% ACCEPTED: 5.11%

% MALE/FEMALE RATIO: 52/48

% UNDERREP. MINORITIES: 14%

APPLICATION DEADLINE: 10/15

APPLICATION NOTIFICATION: Rolling

EARLY APPLICATION DEADLINE: NA

EARLY APPLICATION NOTIFICATION: NA

TRANSFERS ACCEPTED: Yes

ADMISSIONS DEFFERABLE: No

APPLICATION FEE: $75

INTERVIEW TIMEFRAMES: NA

MCAT SCORES: 30.51

GPA: 3.6

IN-STATE TUITION: $27,317

OUT-OF-STATE TUITION: $37,817

TYPE OF SCHOOL: Public

PENNSYLVANIA STATE UNIVERSITY

College of Medicine
Office of Student Affairs
P.O. Box 850
Hershey, PA 17033
Phone: 717-531-8755
Fax: 717-531-625
hmcsaff@psu.edu
www.hmc.psu.edu/college

TOTAL ENROLLMENT: 423

% ACCEPTED: 2.04%

% MALE/FEMALE RATIO: 50/50

% UNDERREP. MINORITIES: 13%

APPLICATION DEADLINE: 11/15

APPLICATION NOTIFICATION: Until Filled

EARLY APPLICATION DEADLINE: 6/1-8/1

EARLY APPLICATION NOTIFICATION: 10/1

TRANSFERS ACCEPTED: Yes

ADMISSIONS DEFFERABLE: Yes

APPLICATION FEE: $40

INTERVIEW TIMEFRAMES: September-March

MCAT SCORES: 28.62

GPA: 3.65

IN-STATE TUITION: $7,349

OUT-OF-STATE TUITION: $7,349

TYPE OF SCHOOL: Private

PONCE SCHOOL OF MEDICINE

P.O. Box 7004
Ponce, PR 00732
Phone: 787-840-2575
Fax: 787-842-0421
admissions@psm.edu
www.psm.edu

TOTAL ENROLLMENT: NA

% ACCEPTED: 15.23%

% MALE/FEMALE RATIO: NA

% UNDERREP. MINORITIES: NA

APPLICATION DEADLINE: 12/15

APPLICATION NOTIFICATION: Rolling

EARLY APPLICATION DEADLINE: 8/1

EARLY APPLICATION NOTIFICATION: 10/5

TRANSFERS ACCEPTED: Yes

ADMISSIONS DEFFERABLE: No

APPLICATION FEE: $100

INTERVIEW TIMEFRAMES: NA

MCAT SCORES: 22

GPA: 3.25

IN-STATE TUITION: $27,065

OUT-OF-STATE TUITION: $27,065

TYPE OF SCHOOL: Private

QUEEN'S UNIVERSITY

School of Medicine
68 Barrie Street
Kingston, ON K7L 3N6
Phone: 613-533-2542
Fax: 613-533-6190
jeb8@post.queensu.ca
meds.queensu.ca

TOTAL ENROLLMENT: 100

% ACCEPTED: 12.61%

% MALE/FEMALE RATIO: 52/48

% UNDERREP. MINORITIES: 2%

APPLICATION DEADLINE: 10/1

APPLICATION NOTIFICATION: 5/31

EARLY APPLICATION DEADLINE: NA

EARLY APPLICATION NOTIFICATION: NA

TRANSFERS ACCEPTED: No

ADMISSIONS DEFFERABLE: Yes

APPLICATION FEE: $250

INTERVIEW TIMEFRAMES: NA

MCAT SCORES: 32.95

GPA: 3.6

IN-STATE TUITION: $13,500

OUT-OF-STATE TUITION: $13,500

TYPE OF SCHOOL: Public

ROSALIND FRANKLIN UNIVERSITY OF MEDICINE AND SCIENCE

Office of Admissions
3333 Green Bay Road North
Chicago, IL 60064
Phone: 847-578-3204
Fax: 847-578-3284
cms.admissions@rosalindfranklin.edu
www.rosalindfranklin.edu

TOTAL ENROLLMENT: 757

% ACCEPTED: 6.90%

% MALE/FEMALE RATIO: 55/45

% UNDERREP. MINORITIES: 6%

APPLICATION DEADLINE: 11/15

APPLICATION NOTIFICATION: 10/15

EARLY APPLICATION DEADLINE: 6/1-8/1

EARLY APPLICATION NOTIFICATION: 10/1

TRANSFERS ACCEPTED: Yes

ADMISSIONS DEFFERABLE: Yes

APPLICATION FEE: $95

INTERVIEW TIMEFRAMES: NA

MCAT SCORES: 29.57

GPA: 3.59

IN-STATE TUITION: $54,720

OUT-OF-STATE TUITION: $54,720

TYPE OF SCHOOL: Private

RUSH UNIVERSITY

Rush Medical College
Office of Admissions, 524 AAC
600 South Paulina
Chicago, IL 60612
Phone: 312-942-6913
Fax: 312-942-2333
rmc_admissions@rush.edu
www.rushu.edu/medcol

TOTAL ENROLLMENT: NA

% ACCEPTED: 14.34%

% MALE/FEMALE RATIO: NA

% UNDERREP. MINORITIES: NA

APPLICATION DEADLINE: 11/1

APPLICATION NOTIFICATION: Rolling

EARLY APPLICATION DEADLINE: 6/1-8/1

EARLY APPLICATION NOTIFICATION: 10/1

TRANSFERS ACCEPTED: No

ADMISSIONS DEFFERABLE: Yes

APPLICATION FEE: $65

INTERVIEW TIMEFRAMES: September-March

MCAT SCORES: 29.5

GPA: 3.5

IN-STATE TUITION: $34,848

OUT-OF-STATE TUITION: $34,848

TYPE OF SCHOOL: Private

SAINT LOUIS UNIVERSITY

School of Medicine
Committee on Admissions
1402 South Grand Blvd., M226
St. Louis, MO 63104
Phone: 314-977-9870
Fax: 314-977-9825
slumd@slu.edu
www.medschool.slu.edu/admissions

TOTAL ENROLLMENT: 616

% ACCEPTED: 1.18%

% MALE/FEMALE RATIO: 53/47

% UNDERREP. MINORITIES: 11%

APPLICATION DEADLINE: 12/15

APPLICATION NOTIFICATION: 10/15

EARLY APPLICATION DEADLINE: 6/1-8/1

EARLY APPLICATION NOTIFICATION: 10/1

TRANSFERS ACCEPTED: Yes

ADMISSIONS DEFFERABLE: Yes

APPLICATION FEE: $100

INTERVIEW TIMEFRAMES: NA

MCAT SCORES: 31.35

GPA: 3.7

IN-STATE TUITION: $50,860

OUT-OF-STATE TUITION: $50,860

TYPE OF SCHOOL: Private

SOUTHERN ILLINOIS UNVERSITY

School of Medicine
P.O. Box 19624
Springfield, IL 62794-9624
Phone: 217-545-6013
Fax: 217-545-5538
admissions@siumed.edu

www.siumed.edu

TOTAL ENROLLMENT: 291

% ACCEPTED: 19.00%

% MALE/FEMALE RATIO: 48/52

% UNDERREP. MINORITIES: 15%

APPLICATION DEADLINE: 11/15

APPLICATION NOTIFICATION: 10/15

EARLY APPLICATION DEADLINE: NA

EARLY APPLICATION NOTIFICATION: NA

TRANSFERS ACCEPTED: Yes

ADMISSIONS DEFFERABLE: Yes

APPLICATION FEE: $50

INTERVIEW TIMEFRAMES: August-April

MCAT SCORES: 26.34

GPA: 3.5

IN-STATE TUITION: $31,962

OUT-OF-STATE TUITION: $68,586

TYPE OF SCHOOL: Public

SPARTAN HEALTH SCIENCES UNIVERSITY

School of Medicine
P.O. Box 324 Vieux Fort
St. Lucia, West Indies
Phone: 758-454-6128
Fax: 758-454-6811
spartanmed@aol.com

www.spartanmed.org

TOTAL ENROLLMENT: 250

% ACCEPTED: 29.40%

% MALE/FEMALE RATIO: 65/35

% UNDERREP. MINORITIES: 90%

APPLICATION DEADLINE: 7/15

APPLICATION NOTIFICATION: 3/15

EARLY APPLICATION DEADLINE: NA

EARLY APPLICATION NOTIFICATION: NA

TRANSFERS ACCEPTED: Yes

ADMISSIONS DEFFERABLE: Yes

APPLICATION FEE: $60

INTERVIEW TIMEFRAMES: NA

MCAT SCORES: NA

GPA: 3.0

IN-STATE TUITION: $13,500

OUT-OF-STATE TUITION: $13,500

TYPE OF SCHOOL: Private

STANFORD UNIVERSITY

School of Medicine
Office of MD Admissions
251 Campus Dr., MSOB XC301
Stanford, CA 94305-5404
Phone: 650-723-6861
Fax: 650-725-7855
mdadmissions@stanford.edu
www.med.stanford.edu

TOTAL ENROLLMENT: 462

% ACCEPTED: 3.42%

% MALE/FEMALE RATIO: 53/47

% UNDERREP. MINORITIES: 22%

APPLICATION DEADLINE: 10/15

APPLICATION NOTIFICATION: Rolling

EARLY APPLICATION DEADLINE: 6/1-8/1

EARLY APPLICATION NOTIFICATION: 10/15

TRANSFERS ACCEPTED: Yes

ADMISSIONS DEFFERABLE: Yes

APPLICATION FEE: $75

INTERVIEW TIMEFRAMES: NA

MCAT SCORES: 33.57

GPA: 3.8

IN-STATE TUITION: $50,716

OUT-OF-STATE TUITION: $50,716

TYPE OF SCHOOL: Private

STATE UNIVERSITY OF NEW YORK

Downstate Medical Center
Office of Admissions
450 Clarkson Avenue
P.O. Box 60M
Brooklyn, NY 11203
Phone: 718-270-2446
Fax: 718-270-7592
admissions@downstate.edu
www.hscbklyn.edu

TOTAL ENROLLMENT: 757

% ACCEPTED: NA

% MALE/FEMALE RATIO: 50/50

% UNDERREP. MINORITIES: 15%

APPLICATION DEADLINE: 12/15

APPLICATION NOTIFICATION: 10/15

EARLY APPLICATION DEADLINE: 6/1-8/1

EARLY APPLICATION NOTIFICATION: 10/1

TRANSFERS ACCEPTED: No

ADMISSIONS DEFFERABLE: Yes

APPLICATION FEE: $65

INTERVIEW TIMEFRAMES: September-April

MCAT SCORES: NA

GPA: NA

IN-STATE TUITION: $11,060

OUT-OF-STATE TUITION: $21,962

TYPE OF SCHOOL: Public

STATE UNIVERSITY OF NEW YORK

Stony Brook University
School of Medicine
Committee on Admissions, Level 4, Rm 147
Health Sciencess
Stony Brook, NY 11794
Phone: 631-444-2113
Fax: 631-444-6032
somadmissions@stonybrook.edu
www.hsc.sunysb.edu/som

TOTAL ENROLLMENT: 447

% ACCEPTED: 13.40%

% MALE/FEMALE RATIO: 53/47

% UNDERREP. MINORITIES: 14%

APPLICATION DEADLINE: 12/15

APPLICATION NOTIFICATION: 10/15

EARLY APPLICATION DEADLINE: 6/1-8/1

EARLY APPLICATION NOTIFICATION: 10/1

TRANSFERS ACCEPTED: Yes

ADMISSIONS DEFFERABLE: Yes

APPLICATION FEE: $75

INTERVIEW TIMEFRAMES: September-March

MCAT SCORES: 24

GPA: 3.6

IN-STATE TUITION: $42,586

OUT-OF-STATE TUITION: $57,286

TYPE OF SCHOOL: Public

STATE UNIVERSITY OF NEW YORK

University at Buffalo
School of Medicine and Biomedical Sciences
131 Beb
Buffalo, NY 14214-3013
Phone: 716-829-3466
Fax: 716-829-3849
jjrosso@buffalo.edu
www.smbs.buffalo.edu

TOTAL ENROLLMENT: 575

% ACCEPTED: 12.91%

% MALE/FEMALE RATIO: 50/50

% UNDERREP. MINORITIES: 7%

APPLICATION DEADLINE: 11/15

APPLICATION NOTIFICATION: 10/15

EARLY APPLICATION DEADLINE: 8/1 Or 8/31

EARLY APPLICATION NOTIFICATION: 10/

TRANSFERS ACCEPTED: No

ADMISSIONS DEFFERABLE: Yes

APPLICATION FEE: $65

INTERVIEW TIMEFRAMES: September-February

MCAT SCORES: 29.13

GPA: 3.57

IN-STATE TUITION: $31,415

OUT-OF-STATE TUITION: $45,615

TYPE OF SCHOOL: Public

STATE UNIVERSITY OF NEW YORK

Upstate Medical University
College of Medicine
Office of Student Admissions
766 Irving Avenue
Syracuse, NY 13210
Phone: 315-464-4570
Fax: 315-464-8867
admiss@upstate.edu
www.upstate.edu

TOTAL ENROLLMENT: 652

% ACCEPTED: 12.30%

% MALE/FEMALE RATIO: 54/46

% UNDERREP. MINORITIES: 8%

APPLICATION DEADLINE: 12/1

APPLICATION NOTIFICATION: 5/1

EARLY APPLICATION DEADLINE: 8/1

EARLY APPLICATION NOTIFICATION: 10/1

TRANSFERS ACCEPTED: Yes

ADMISSIONS DEFFERABLE: Yes

APPLICATION FEE: $100

INTERVIEW TIMEFRAMES: September-March

MCAT SCORES: 29.59

GPA: 3.54

IN-STATE TUITION: $21,890

OUT-OF-STATE TUITION: $36,590

TYPE OF SCHOOL: Public

TEMPLE UNIVERSITY

School of Medicine
3340 North Broad Street, SFC Suite 305
Philadelphia, PA 19140
Phone: 215-707-3656
Fax: 215-707-6932
medadmissions@temple.edu
www.template.edu/medicine

TOTAL ENROLLMENT: NA

% ACCEPTED: 11.90%

% MALE/FEMALE RATIO: NA

% UNDERREP. MINORITIES: NA

APPLICATION DEADLINE: 12/15

APPLICATION NOTIFICATION: 10/15

EARLY APPLICATION DEADLINE: 8/1

EARLY APPLICATION NOTIFICATION: 10/1

TRANSFERS ACCEPTED: Yes

ADMISSIONS DEFFERABLE: Yes

APPLICATION FEE: $70

INTERVIEW TIMEFRAMES: September-April

MCAT SCORES: 30

GPA: 3.59

IN-STATE TUITION: $49,483

OUT-OF-STATE TUITION: $57,063

TYPE OF SCHOOL: Private

TEXAS A&M UNIVERSITY SYSTEM

Health Science Center
College of Medicine
159 Joe H. Reynolds MB
College Station, TX 77843
Phone: 979-845-7743
Fax: 979-845-5533
admissions@medicine.tamhsc.edu

www.medicine.tamhsc.edu

TOTAL ENROLLMENT: 300

% ACCEPTED: 8.92%

% MALE/FEMALE RATIO: 52/48

% UNDERREP. MINORITIES: 14%

APPLICATION DEADLINE: 10/15

APPLICATION NOTIFICATION: 11/15

EARLY APPLICATION DEADLINE: NA

EARLY APPLICATION NOTIFICATION: NA

TRANSFERS ACCEPTED: Yes

ADMISSIONS DEFFERABLE: Yes

APPLICATION FEE: $45

INTERVIEW TIMEFRAMES: August-December

MCAT SCORES: 27.7

GPA: 3.73

IN-STATE TUITION: $23,314

OUT-OF-STATE TUITION: $35,214

TYPE OF SCHOOL: Public

TEXAS TECH UNIVERSITY

TTU Health Sciences Center
School of Medicine
3601 4th Street, 2B116
Lubbock, TX 79430
Phone: 806-743-2297
Fax: 806-743-2725
trevor.yates@ttuhsc.edu

www.ttuhsc.edu

TOTAL ENROLLMENT: 490

% ACCEPTED: 10.53%

% MALE/FEMALE RATIO: 44/56

% UNDERREP. MINORITIES: 22%

APPLICATION DEADLINE: 12/1

APPLICATION NOTIFICATION: Rolling

EARLY APPLICATION DEADLINE: 8/1

EARLY APPLICATION NOTIFICATION: 10/1

TRANSFERS ACCEPTED: Yes

ADMISSIONS DEFFERABLE: Yes

APPLICATION FEE: $40

INTERVIEW TIMEFRAMES: September-January

MCAT SCORES: 28.7

GPA: 305

IN-STATE TUITION: $21,151

OUT-OF-STATE TUITION: $35,251

TYPE OF SCHOOL: Public

THOMAS JEFFERSON UNIVERSITY

Jefferson Medical College
1015 Walnut Street, Room 110
Philadelphia, PA 19107
Phone: 215-955-6983
Fax: 215-955-5151
jmc.admissions@jefferson.edu
www.jefferson.edu/jmc/

TOTAL ENROLLMENT: 935

% ACCEPTED: 6.71%

% MALE/FEMALE RATIO: 51/49

% UNDERREP. MINORITIES: 26%

APPLICATION DEADLINE: 11/15

APPLICATION NOTIFICATION: Rolling

EARLY APPLICATION DEADLINE: 6/1-8/1

EARLY APPLICATION NOTIFICATION: 10/1

TRANSFERS ACCEPTED: Yes

ADMISSIONS DEFFERABLE: Yes

APPLICATION FEE: $80

INTERVIEW TIMEFRAMES: September-March

MCAT SCORES: 30.6

GPA: 3.6

IN-STATE TUITION: $59,805

OUT-OF-STATE TUITION: $59,805

TYPE OF SCHOOL: Private

TUFTS UNIVERSITY

School of Medicine
Office of Admissions
136 Harrison Avenue, Stearns 1
Boston, MA 02111
Phone: 617-636-6571
sgp@cor.cdm.nemc.
www.tufts.edu/med

TOTAL ENROLLMENT: 695

% ACCEPTED: 5.71%

% MALE/FEMALE RATIO: 54/46

% UNDERREP. MINORITIES: 11%

APPLICATION DEADLINE: 11/1

APPLICATION NOTIFICATION: Rolling

EARLY APPLICATION DEADLINE: 8/1

EARLY APPLICATION NOTIFICATION: 10/1

TRANSFERS ACCEPTED: Yes

ADMISSIONS DEFFERABLE: Yes

APPLICATION FEE: $95

INTERVIEW TIMEFRAMES: November-March

MCAT SCORES: 30.7

GPA: 3.5

IN-STATE TUITION: $53,622

OUT-OF-STATE TUITION: $53,622

TYPE OF SCHOOL: Private

TULANE UNIVERSITY

School of Medicine
Office of Admissions
1430 Tulane Avenue, Sl67
New Orleans, LA 70112
Phone: 504-588-5187
Fax: 504-599-6735
medsch@tmcpop.tmc.tulane.edu

www.mcl.tulane.edu

TOTAL ENROLLMENT: 599

% ACCEPTED: NA

% MALE/FEMALE RATIO: 58/42

% UNDERREP. MINORITIES: 12%

APPLICATION DEADLINE: 12/15

APPLICATION NOTIFICATION: 10/15

EARLY APPLICATION DEADLINE: 6/1-8/1

EARLY APPLICATION NOTIFICATION: 10/1

TRANSFERS ACCEPTED: Yes

ADMISSIONS DEFFERABLE: Yes

APPLICATION FEE: $95

INTERVIEW TIMEFRAMES: September-February

MCAT SCORES: 31

GPA: 3.5

IN-STATE TUITION: NA

OUT-OF-STATE TUITION: NA

TYPE OF SCHOOL: Private

UNIFORMED SERVICES UNIVERSITY OF THE HEALTH SCIENCES

F. Edward Hebert School of Medicine
4301 Jones Bridge Road, Room A1041
Bethesda, MD 20814
Phone: 301-295-3101 Or 800-722-1743
Fax: 301-295-3545
admissions@usuhs.mil

www.usuhs.mil

TOTAL ENROLLMENT: 665

% ACCEPTED: 15.30%

% MALE/FEMALE RATIO: 69/31

% UNDERREP. MINORITIES: 20%

APPLICATION DEADLINE: 11/1

APPLICATION NOTIFICATION: Rolling

EARLY APPLICATION DEADLINE: NA

EARLY APPLICATION NOTIFICATION: NA

TRANSFERS ACCEPTED: No

ADMISSIONS DEFFERABLE: Yes

APPLICATION FEE: NA

INTERVIEW TIMEFRAMES: September-February

MCAT SCORES: 29.2

GPA: 3.5

IN-STATE TUITION: NA

OUT-OF-STATE TUITION: NA

TYPE OF SCHOOL: Public

UNIVERSIDAD CENTRAL DE CARIBE

Universidad Central De Caribe
Call Box 60-327
Bayamon, PR 00960-6032
Phone: 787-798-3001 Ext. 2403
Fax: 787-269-7550
lcordero@uccaribe.edu

www.uccaribe.edu

TOTAL ENROLLMENT: 240

% ACCEPTED: 15.63%

% MALE/FEMALE RATIO: 49/51

% UNDERREP. MINORITIES: 5%

APPLICATION DEADLINE: 12/15

APPLICATION NOTIFICATION: 2/15

EARLY APPLICATION DEADLINE: NA

EARLY APPLICATION NOTIFICATION: NA

TRANSFERS ACCEPTED: Yes

ADMISSIONS DEFFERABLE: No

APPLICATION FEE: $50

INTERVIEW TIMEFRAMES: NA

MCAT SCORES: 21.06

GPA: 3.31

IN-STATE TUITION: $32,290

OUT-OF-STATE TUITION: $32,290

TYPE OF SCHOOL: Private

UNIVERSITE LAVAL

Faculté De Médicine
Pavillon Vandry
U. Laval Foy
QC G1K 7P4
Phone: 418-656-2131
Fax: 418-656-2733
guy.labrecque@fmed.ulaval.ca

www.fmed.ulaval.ca

TOTAL ENROLLMENT: NA

% ACCEPTED: 13.80%

% MALE/FEMALE RATIO: NA

% UNDERREP. MINORITIES: NA

APPLICATION DEADLINE: 3/1

APPLICATION NOTIFICATION: 5/15

EARLY APPLICATION DEADLINE: NA

EARLY APPLICATION NOTIFICATION: NA

TRANSFERS ACCEPTED: No

ADMISSIONS DEFFERABLE: No

APPLICATION FEE: $30

INTERVIEW TIMEFRAMES: NA

MCAT SCORES: NA

GPA: NA

IN-STATE TUITION: $2,164

OUT-OF-STATE TUITION: $8,127

TYPE OF SCHOOL: Public

UNIVERSITY OF ALABAMA AT BIRMINGHAM

School of Medicine
Medical Student Services, Vh 100
1530 Third Avenue South
Birmingham, AL 35294-0019
Phone: 205-934-2433
Fax: 205-934-8740
medschool@uab.edu

www.uab.edu/uasom

TOTAL ENROLLMENT: 685

% ACCEPTED: 12.30%

% MALE/FEMALE RATIO: 59/41

% UNDERREP. MINORITIES: 22%

APPLICATION DEADLINE: 11/1

APPLICATION NOTIFICATION: 11/15

EARLY APPLICATION DEADLINE: 8/1

EARLY APPLICATION NOTIFICATION: 10/1

TRANSFERS ACCEPTED: Yes

ADMISSIONS DEFFERABLE: Yes

APPLICATION FEE: $70

INTERVIEW TIMEFRAMES: NA

MCAT SCORES: 30.3

GPA: 3.72

IN-STATE TUITION: $32,411

OUT-OF-STATE TUITION: $56,733

TYPE OF SCHOOL: Public

UNIVERSITY OF ALBERTA

Faculty of Medicine and Dentistry
2-45 Medical Sciences Building
Edmonton, AB T6G 2H7
Phone: 780-492-6350
Fax: 780-492-7303
dean@ualberta.ca

www.med.ualberta.ca

TOTAL ENROLLMENT: NA

% ACCEPTED: NA

% MALE/FEMALE RATIO: NA

% UNDERREP. MINORITIES: NA

APPLICATION DEADLINE: 1/31

APPLICATION NOTIFICATION: NA

EARLY APPLICATION DEADLINE: NA

EARLY APPLICATION NOTIFICATION: NA

TRANSFERS ACCEPTED: NA

ADMISSIONS DEFFERABLE: Yes

APPLICATION FEE: $60

INTERVIEW TIMEFRAMES: February-March

MCAT SCORES: 31.8

GPA: NA

IN-STATE TUITION: $12,966

OUT-OF-STATE TUITION: NA

TYPE OF SCHOOL: Public

UNIVERSITY OF ARIZONA

College of Medicine
Admissions Office, Room 2106
P.O. Box 245075
Tucson, AZ 85724
Phone: 520-626-6214
Fax: 520-626-4884
admissions@medicine.arizona.edu
www.medicine.arizona.edu

TOTAL ENROLLMENT: 406

% ACCEPTED: 8.32%

% MALE/FEMALE RATIO: 52/48

% UNDERREP. MINORITIES: 15%

APPLICATION DEADLINE: 11/1

APPLICATION NOTIFICATION: 1/30

EARLY APPLICATION DEADLINE: NA

EARLY APPLICATION NOTIFICATION: NA

TRANSFERS ACCEPTED: No

ADMISSIONS DEFFERABLE: Yes

APPLICATION FEE: $75

INTERVIEW TIMEFRAMES: September-March

MCAT SCORES: NA

GPA: NA

IN-STATE TUITION: $7,932

OUT-OF-STATE TUITION: NA

TYPE OF SCHOOL: Public

UNIVERSITY OF ARKANSAS FOR MEDICAL SCIENCES

College of Medicine
4301 West Markham Street, Slot 551
Little Rock, AR 72205-7199
Phone: 501-686-5354
Fax: 501-68-5873
southtomg@uams.edu
www.uams.edu/com

TOTAL ENROLLMENT: 576

% ACCEPTED: 25.33%

% MALE/FEMALE RATIO: 56/44

% UNDERREP. MINORITIES: 10%

APPLICATION DEADLINE: 11/1

APPLICATION NOTIFICATION: 2/15

EARLY APPLICATION DEADLINE: NA

EARLY APPLICATION NOTIFICATION: NA

TRANSFERS ACCEPTED: Yes

ADMISSIONS DEFFERABLE: Yes

APPLICATION FEE: $100

INTERVIEW TIMEFRAMES: October-January

MCAT SCORES: 27

GPA: 3.6

IN-STATE TUITION: $13,242

OUT-OF-STATE TUITION: $24,884

TYPE OF SCHOOL: Public

University of British Columbia

Faculty of Medicine
317-2194 Health Sciences Hall
British Columbia, BC V6T 1Z3
Phone: 604-822-2421
Fax: 604-822-6061
admissions.md@ubc.ca
www.med.ubc.ca

Total Enrollment: 120

% Accepted: NA

% Male/Female Ratio: NA

% Underrep. Minorities: NA

Application Deadline: 10/1

Application Notification: 3/1

Early Application Deadline: NA

Early Application Notification: NA

Transfers Accepted: Yes

Admissions Defferable: Yes

Application Fee: $105

Interview Timeframes: NA

MCAT Scores: 30

GPA: NA

In-state Tuition: $5,456

Out-of-state Tuition: NA

Type of School: Public

University of Calgary

Faculty of Medicine
3330 Hospital Driver Northwest
Alberta, T2N 4N1
Phone: 403-220-4262
Fax: NA

Total Enrollment: 234

% Accepted: NA

% Male/Female Ratio: 48/52

% Underrep. Minorities: NA

Application Deadline: 11/15

Application Notification: 4/14

Early Application Deadline: NA

Early Application Notification: NA

Transfers Accepted: Yes

Admissions Defferable: Yes

Application Fee: $65

Interview Timeframes: NA

MCAT Scores: 30.92

GPA: 3.5

In-state Tuition: $8,052

Out-of-state Tuition: $31,533

Type of School: Public

UNIVERSITY OF CALIFORNIA—DAVIS

School of Medicine
1 Shields Avenue
Davis, CA 95616-8661
Phone: 530-752-2717
Fax: 530-754-6252
medadmsinfo@ucdavis.edu

www.som.ucdavis.edu

TOTAL ENROLLMENT: 403

% ACCEPTED: 5.00%

% MALE/FEMALE RATIO: 52/48

% UNDERREP. MINORITIES: 14%

APPLICATION DEADLINE: 11/1

APPLICATION NOTIFICATION: 10/1

EARLY APPLICATION DEADLINE: NA

EARLY APPLICATION NOTIFICATION: NA

TRANSFERS ACCEPTED: Yes

ADMISSIONS DEFFERABLE: Yes

APPLICATION FEE: NA

INTERVIEW TIMEFRAMES: October-April

MCAT SCORES: 31

GPA: 3.61

IN-STATE TUITION: $33,184

OUT-OF-STATE TUITION: $45,429

TYPE OF SCHOOL: Public

UNIVERSITY OF CALIFORNIA—IRVINE

College of Medicine
Medical Education Building 802, Room 100
Irvine, CA 92697-4089
Phone: 949-824-5388
Fax: 949-824-2485
medadmit@uci.edu

www.ucihs.edu/admissions

TOTAL ENROLLMENT: 372

% ACCEPTED: 7.18%

% MALE/FEMALE RATIO: 54/46

% UNDERREP. MINORITIES: 8%

APPLICATION DEADLINE: 11/1

APPLICATION NOTIFICATION: Rolling

EARLY APPLICATION DEADLINE: NA

EARLY APPLICATION NOTIFICATION: NA

TRANSFERS ACCEPTED: No

ADMISSIONS DEFFERABLE: Yes

APPLICATION FEE: $60

INTERVIEW TIMEFRAMES: NA

MCAT SCORES: 32

GPA: 3.7

IN-STATE TUITION: NA

OUT-OF-STATE TUITION: $41,159

TYPE OF SCHOOL: Public

UNIVERSITY OF CALIFORNIA— LOS ANGELES

David Geffen School of Medicine at UCLA
Center for Health Sciences
Los Angeles, CA 90095-1720
Phone: 310-825-6081
Fax: 310-825-6081
somadmiss@mednet.ucla.edu

www.medstudent.ucla.edu

TOTAL ENROLLMENT: 674

% ACCEPTED: NA

% MALE/FEMALE RATIO: 58/42

% UNDERREP. MINORITIES: 30%

APPLICATION DEADLINE: 11/1

APPLICATION NOTIFICATION: 1/15

EARLY APPLICATION DEADLINE: NA

EARLY APPLICATION NOTIFICATION: NA

TRANSFERS ACCEPTED: Yes

ADMISSIONS DEFFERABLE: Yes

APPLICATION FEE: $40

INTERVIEW TIMEFRAMES: November-May

MCAT SCORES: NA

GPA: NA

IN-STATE TUITION: $33,533

OUT-OF-STATE TUITION: $45,778

TYPE OF SCHOOL: Public

UNIVERSITY OF CALIFORNIA— SAN DIEGO

School of Medicine
9500 Gilman Drive, MC 0621
La Jolla, CA 92093-0621
Phone: 858-534-3880
Fax: 858-534-5282
somadmissions@ucsd.edu

www.meded.ucsd.edu/admissions

TOTAL ENROLLMENT: 503

% ACCEPTED: 6.00%

% MALE/FEMALE RATIO: 51/49

% UNDERREP. MINORITIES: 18%

APPLICATION DEADLINE: 11/1

APPLICATION NOTIFICATION: 10/15

EARLY APPLICATION DEADLINE: NA

EARLY APPLICATION NOTIFICATION: NA

TRANSFERS ACCEPTED: No

ADMISSIONS DEFFERABLE: Yes

APPLICATION FEE: $60

INTERVIEW TIMEFRAMES: October-May

MCAT SCORES: 32.99

GPA: 3.73

IN-STATE TUITION: $31,706

OUT-OF-STATE TUITION: $34,188

TYPE OF SCHOOL: Public

UNIVERSITY OF CALIFORNIA—SAN FRANCISCO

School of Medicine
School of Medicine Admissions, C-200
P.O. Box 0408
San Francisco, CA 94143-0408
Phone: 415-476-4044
Fax: 415-476-5490
admissions@medsch.ucsf.edu
www.medschool.ucsf.edu/admissions

TOTAL ENROLLMENT: 600

% ACCEPTED: 4.90%

% MALE/FEMALE RATIO: 44/56

% UNDERREP. MINORITIES: 18%

APPLICATION DEADLINE: 11/1

APPLICATION NOTIFICATION: Rolling

EARLY APPLICATION DEADLINE: NA

EARLY APPLICATION NOTIFICATION: NA

TRANSFERS ACCEPTED: No

ADMISSIONS DEFFERABLE: Yes

APPLICATION FEE: $60

INTERVIEW TIMEFRAMES: September-March

MCAT SCORES: 33.8

GPA: 3.79

IN-STATE TUITION: NA

OUT-OF-STATE TUITION: $54,478

TYPE OF SCHOOL: Public

UNIVERSITY OF CHICAGO

Pritzker School of Medicine
Office of Medical Education, BSLC 104W
924 East Fifty-seventh Street
Chicago, IL 60637-5416
Phone: 773-702-1937
Fax: 773-834-5412
pritzkeradmissions@bsd.uchicago.edu
www.pritzker.bsd.uchicago.edu

TOTAL ENROLLMENT: 432

% ACCEPTED: 7.23%

% MALE/FEMALE RATIO: 48/52

% UNDERREP. MINORITIES: 15%

APPLICATION DEADLINE: 10/15

APPLICATION NOTIFICATION: Rolling

EARLY APPLICATION DEADLINE: 8/1

EARLY APPLICATION NOTIFICATION: 10/1

TRANSFERS ACCEPTED: Yes

ADMISSIONS DEFFERABLE: Yes

APPLICATION FEE: $75

INTERVIEW TIMEFRAMES: September-March

MCAT SCORES: 32.8

GPA: 3.74

IN-STATE TUITION: $52,763

OUT-OF-STATE TUITION: $52,763

TYPE OF SCHOOL: Private

UNIVERSITY OF CINCINNATI

College of Medicine
Office of Admissions
P.O. Box 670552
Cincinnati, OH 45267-0552
Phone: 513-558-7314
Fax: 513-558-1165
comadmis@ucmail.uc.edu

www.med.uc.edu

TOTAL ENROLLMENT: 629

% ACCEPTED: 11.54%

% MALE/FEMALE RATIO: 55/45

% UNDERREP. MINORITIES: 13%

APPLICATION DEADLINE: 11/15

APPLICATION NOTIFICATION: Rolling

EARLY APPLICATION DEADLINE: 6/1-8/1

EARLY APPLICATION NOTIFICATION: 10/1

TRANSFERS ACCEPTED: Yes

ADMISSIONS DEFFERABLE: Yes

APPLICATION FEE: $25

INTERVIEW TIMEFRAMES: October 15-May 15

MCAT SCORES: 30.3

GPA: 3.59

IN-STATE TUITION: $41,787

OUT-OF-STATE TUITION: $59,211

TYPE OF SCHOOL: Public

UNIVERSITY OF COLORADO

School of Medicine
Medical School Admissions
4200 East Ninth Avenue, C-297
Denver, CO 80262
Phone: 303-315-7361
Fax: 303-315-1614
somadmin@uchsc.edu

www.uchsc.edu/som/admissions

TOTAL ENROLLMENT: 547

% ACCEPTED: 9.74%

% MALE/FEMALE RATIO: 54/46

% UNDERREP. MINORITIES: 15%

APPLICATION DEADLINE: 11/1

APPLICATION NOTIFICATION: Rolling

EARLY APPLICATION DEADLINE: NA

EARLY APPLICATION NOTIFICATION: NA

TRANSFERS ACCEPTED: No

ADMISSIONS DEFFERABLE: Yes

APPLICATION FEE: $100

INTERVIEW TIMEFRAMES: September-March

MCAT SCORES: 31.86

GPA: 3.68

IN-STATE TUITION: $23,828

OUT-OF-STATE TUITION: $75,401

TYPE OF SCHOOL: Public

University of Connecticut

School of Medicine
Medical Student Affairs
263 Farmington Avenue, Rm AG-062
Farmington, CT 06030-1905
Phone: 860-679-3874
Fax: 860-679-1282
sanford@nso1.uchc.edu
www.uchc.edu

Total Enrollment: 313

% Accepted: 7.20%

% Male/Female Ratio: 37/63

% Underrep. Minorities: 33%

Application Deadline: 12/15

Application Notification: 10/15

Early Application Deadline: 6/1-8/1

Early Application Notification: 10/1

Transfers Accepted: Yes

Admissions Defferable: Yes

Application Fee: $75

Interview Timeframes: August-April

MCAT Scores: 30.7

GPA: 3.66

In-state Tuition: $43,445

Out-of-state Tuition: $63,685

Type of School: Public

University of Florida

College of Medicine
P.O. Box 100216
J. Hillis Miller Health Center
1600 Southwest Archer Road
Gainesville, FL 32610-0216
Phone: 352-392-4569
Fax: 352-846-0622
admissions@mail.med.ufl.edu
www.med.ufl.edu

Total Enrollment: 458

% Accepted: 9.50%

% Male/Female Ratio: 49/51

% Underrep. Minorities: 16%

Application Deadline: 12/1

Application Notification: Rolling

Early Application Deadline: NA

Early Application Notification: NA

Transfers Accepted: Yes

Admissions Defferable: Yes

Application Fee: $30

Interview Timeframes: September-March

MCAT Scores: 31.25

GPA: 3.7

In-state Tuition: $28,822

Out-of-state Tuition: $59,719

Type of School: Public

UNIVERSITY OF HAWAII

John A. Burns School of Medicine (Jabsom)
651 Llalo Street
Honolulu, HI 96813
Phone: 808-692-1000
Fax: 808-692-1251
mnishiki@hawaii.edu

jabsom.hawaii.edu

TOTAL ENROLLMENT: 260

% ACCEPTED: NA

% MALE/FEMALE RATIO: 40/60

% UNDERREP. MINORITIES: 17%

APPLICATION DEADLINE: 11/1

APPLICATION NOTIFICATION: 10/15

EARLY APPLICATION DEADLINE: 6/1-8/1

EARLY APPLICATION NOTIFICATION: 10/1

TRANSFERS ACCEPTED: Yes

ADMISSIONS DEFFERABLE: Yes

APPLICATION FEE: $50

INTERVIEW TIMEFRAMES: October-March

MCAT SCORES: 29

GPA: 3.6

IN-STATE TUITION: $20,574

OUT-OF-STATE TUITION: $37,190

TYPE OF SCHOOL: Public

UNIVERSITY OF ILLINOIS AT CHICAGO

UIC College of Medicine
808 South Wood Street
Room 165 CME, M/C 783
Chicago, IL 60612
Phone: 312-996-5635
Fax: 312-996-6693
medadmit@uic.edu

www.medicine.uic.edu

TOTAL ENROLLMENT: 1242

% ACCEPTED: 14.30%

% MALE/FEMALE RATIO: 59/41

% UNDERREP. MINORITIES: 21&%

APPLICATION DEADLINE: 12/31

APPLICATION NOTIFICATION: 6/1

EARLY APPLICATION DEADLINE: 6/1-8/1

EARLY APPLICATION NOTIFICATION: 10/1

TRANSFERS ACCEPTED: Yes

ADMISSIONS DEFFERABLE: Yes

APPLICATION FEE: $40

INTERVIEW TIMEFRAMES: September-April

MCAT SCORES: 28

GPA: 3.5

IN-STATE TUITION: NA

OUT-OF-STATE TUITION: NA

TYPE OF SCHOOL: Public

UNIVERSITY OF IOWA

Roy J. & Lucille A. Carver
  College of Medicine
100 Medicine Administration Building
Iowa City, IA 52242
Phone: 319-335-8052
Fax: 319-335-8049
medical-admission@uiowa.edu
www.medicine.uiowa.edu/osac/admissions

TOTAL ENROLLMENT: 562

% ACCEPTED: 11.94%

% MALE/FEMALE RATIO: 53/47

% UNDERREP. MINORITIES: 25%

APPLICATION DEADLINE: 11/1

APPLICATION NOTIFICATION: Rolling

EARLY APPLICATION DEADLINE: 6/1-8/1

EARLY APPLICATION NOTIFICATION: 10/1

TRANSFERS ACCEPTED: No

ADMISSIONS DEFFERABLE: Yes

APPLICATION FEE: $50

INTERVIEW TIMEFRAMES: NA

MCAT SCORES: 30.7

GPA: 3.72

IN-STATE TUITION: $22,908

OUT-OF-STATE TUITION: $42,114

TYPE OF SCHOOL: Public

UNIVERSITY OF KANSAS

School of Medicine
3901 Rainbow Boulevard
3040 Murphy Building, Mail Stop 1049
Kansas City, KS 66160
Phone: 913-588-5245
Fax: 913-588-5259
premedinfo@kumc.edu
www.kumc.edu/som/som.html

TOTAL ENROLLMENT: 700

% ACCEPTED: 14.50%

% MALE/FEMALE RATIO: 55/45

% UNDERREP. MINORITIES: 14%

APPLICATION DEADLINE: 10/15

APPLICATION NOTIFICATION: 3/31

EARLY APPLICATION DEADLINE: 7/1/2007 (Recommended)

EARLY APPLICATION NOTIFICATION: 10/1

TRANSFERS ACCEPTED: Yes

ADMISSIONS DEFFERABLE: Yes

APPLICATION FEE: NA

INTERVIEW TIMEFRAMES: October-March

MCAT SCORES: 28.6

GPA: 3.66

IN-STATE TUITION: $31,496

OUT-OF-STATE TUITION: $47,250

TYPE OF SCHOOL: Public

UNIVERSITY OF KENTUCKY

College of Medicine
MN118 UKMC
800 Rose Street
Lexington, KY 40536-0298
Phone: 859-323-6161
Fax: 859-257-3633
kymedap@uky.edu

www.comed.uky.edu/medicine

TOTAL ENROLLMENT: 400

% ACCEPTED: NA

% MALE/FEMALE RATIO: 57/43

% UNDERREP. MINORITIES: 6%

APPLICATION DEADLINE: 11/1

APPLICATION NOTIFICATION: Rolling

EARLY APPLICATION DEADLINE: 6/1-8/1

EARLY APPLICATION NOTIFICATION: 10/1

TRANSFERS ACCEPTED: Yes

ADMISSIONS DEFFERABLE: Yes

APPLICATION FEE: $50

INTERVIEW TIMEFRAMES: September-March

MCAT SCORES: 29.4

GPA: 3.64

IN-STATE TUITION: $31,730

OUT-OF-STATE TUITION: $50,704

TYPE OF SCHOOL: Public

UNIVERSITY OF LOUISVILLE

School of Medicine
Abell Administration Center, Rm 413
323 East Chestnut Street
Louisville, KY 40202
Phone: 502-852-5193
Fax: 502-852-0302
medadm@louiseville.edu

www.louiseville.edu

TOTAL ENROLLMENT: 588

% ACCEPTED: 14.34%

% MALE/FEMALE RATIO: 56/44

% UNDERREP. MINORITIES: 16%

APPLICATION DEADLINE: 10/15

APPLICATION NOTIFICATION: Rolling

EARLY APPLICATION DEADLINE: 6/1-8/1

EARLY APPLICATION NOTIFICATION: 10/1

TRANSFERS ACCEPTED: Yes

ADMISSIONS DEFFERABLE: Yes

APPLICATION FEE: $75

INTERVIEW TIMEFRAMES: September-February

MCAT SCORES: 28.44

GPA: 3.6

IN-STATE TUITION: $28,724

OUT-OF-STATE TUITION: $51,090

TYPE OF SCHOOL: Public

UNIVERSITY OF MANITOBA

270-727 Mcdermot Avenue
Winnipeg, MB R3E 0W3
Phone: 204-789-3499
Fax: 204-78-3929
registrar_med@umanitoba.ca
www.umanitoba.ca/medicine

TOTAL ENROLLMENT: 362

% ACCEPTED: 19.40%

% MALE/FEMALE RATIO: 53/47

% UNDERREP. MINORITIES: 5%

APPLICATION DEADLINE: 10/2

APPLICATION NOTIFICATION: 5/15

EARLY APPLICATION DEADLINE: NA

EARLY APPLICATION NOTIFICATION: NA

TRANSFERS ACCEPTED: Yes

ADMISSIONS DEFFERABLE: Yes

APPLICATION FEE: $75

INTERVIEW TIMEFRAMES: NA

MCAT SCORES: 30.92

GPA: 4.0

IN-STATE TUITION: $17,595

OUT-OF-STATE TUITION: $17,595

TYPE OF SCHOOL: Public

UNIVERSITY OF MARYLAND

School of Medicine
Suite 190
685 West Baltimore Street
Baltimore, MD 21201-1559
Phone: 410-706-7478
Fax: 410-706-0467
admissions@som.umaryland.edu
www.medschool.umaryland.edu

TOTAL ENROLLMENT: 604

% ACCEPTED: 8.40%

% MALE/FEMALE RATIO: 40/60

% UNDERREP. MINORITIES: 13%

APPLICATION DEADLINE: 11/1

APPLICATION NOTIFICATION: 10/1

EARLY APPLICATION DEADLINE: 8/1

EARLY APPLICATION NOTIFICATION: 10/1

TRANSFERS ACCEPTED: Yes

ADMISSIONS DEFFERABLE: Yes

APPLICATION FEE: $70

INTERVIEW TIMEFRAMES: Start In October

MCAT SCORES: 30.7

GPA: 3.66

IN-STATE TUITION: $33,782

OUT-OF-STATE TUITION: $49,649

TYPE OF SCHOOL: Public

UNIVERSITY OF MASSACHUSETTS

Medical School
Associate Dean for Admissions
55 Lake Avenue North
Worcester, MA 01655
Phone: 508-856-2323
Fax: 506-856-3629
admissions@umassmed.edu
www.umassmed.edu/som/admissions

TOTAL ENROLLMENT: 425

% ACCEPTED: NA

% MALE/FEMALE RATIO: 49/51

% UNDERREP. MINORITIES: 7%

APPLICATION DEADLINE: 11/1

APPLICATION NOTIFICATION: 5/15

EARLY APPLICATION DEADLINE: 6/1-8/1

EARLY APPLICATION NOTIFICATION: 10/1

TRANSFERS ACCEPTED: Yes

ADMISSIONS DEFFERABLE: Yes

APPLICATION FEE: $50

INTERVIEW TIMEFRAMES: October-March

MCAT SCORES: NA

GPA: NA

IN-STATE TUITION: $10,647

OUT-OF-STATE TUITION: NA

TYPE OF SCHOOL: Public

UNIVERSITY OF MEDICINE A[nd] DENTISTRY OF NEW JERSE[y]

New Jersey Medical School
185 South Orange Avenue
Medical Science Building, Rm C-653
Newark, NJ 07103
Phone: 973-972-4631
Fax: 973-972-7986
njmsadmiss@umdnj.edu
www.njms.umdnj.edu

TOTAL ENROLLMENT: 695

% ACCEPTED: 4.20%

% MALE/FEMALE RATIO: 51/49

% UNDERREP. MINORITIES: 32%

APPLICATION DEADLINE: 6/1-12/1

APPLICATION NOTIFICATION: 10/15

EARLY APPLICATION DEADLINE: 6/1-8/1

EARLY APPLICATION NOTIFICATION: 10/1

TRANSFERS ACCEPTED: Yes

ADMISSIONS DEFFERABLE: Yes

APPLICATION FEE: $75

INTERVIEW TIMEFRAMES: NA

MCAT SCORES: 29

GPA: 3.61

IN-STATE TUITION: $22,200

OUT-OF-STATE TUITION: $34,282

TYPE OF SCHOOL: Public

University of Medicine and Dentistry of New Jersey

Robert Wood Johnson Medical School
Office of Admissions
675 Hoes Lane
Piscataway, NJ 08854
Phone: 732-235-4576
Fax: 732-235-5078
rwjapadm@umdnj.edu
www.rwjms.umdnj.edu

Total Enrollment: 642

% Accepted: 12.30%

% Male/Female Ratio: 47/53

% Underrep. Minorities: 16%

Application Deadline: 12/1

Application Notification: Rolling

Early Application Deadline: 6/1-8/1

Early Application Notification: 10/1

Transfers Accepted: Yes

Admissions Defferable: Yes

Application Fee: $75

Interview Timeframes: NA

MCAT Scores: 30.2

GPA: 3.62

In-state Tuition: $36,186

Out-of-state Tuition: $48,268

Type of School: Public

University of Miami

Miller School of Medicine
Admissions R-159
P.O. Box 016159
Miami, FL 33101
Phone: 305-243-6791
Fax: 305-243-6548
med.admissions@miami.edu
www.miami.edu/medical-admissions

Total Enrollment: 615

% Accepted: 6.34%

% Male/Female Ratio: 48/52

% Underrep. Minorities: 7%

Application Deadline: 12/1

Application Notification: 10/15

Early Application Deadline: NA

Early Application Notification: NA

Transfers Accepted: No

Admissions Defferable: Yes

Application Fee: $65

Interview Timeframes: August-April

MCAT Scores: 29.3

GPA: 3.71

In-state Tuition: $30,648

Out-of-state Tuition: $39,854

Type of School: Private

UNIVERSITY OF MICHIGAN

Medical School
Admissions Office
M4130 Medical Science 1 Building
Ann Arbor, MI 48109
Phone: 313-764-6317
Fax: 313-936-3510
pibs@umich.edu

www.med.umich.edu/medschool

TOTAL ENROLLMENT: 177

% ACCEPTED: NA

% MALE/FEMALE RATIO: 51/49

% UNDERREP. MINORITIES: 15%

APPLICATION DEADLINE: 11/15

APPLICATION NOTIFICATION: Rolling

EARLY APPLICATION DEADLINE: 6/1-8/1

EARLY APPLICATION NOTIFICATION: 10/1

TRANSFERS ACCEPTED: No

ADMISSIONS DEFFERABLE: Yes

APPLICATION FEE: $50

INTERVIEW TIMEFRAMES: September-March

MCAT SCORES: NA

GPA: 3.72

IN-STATE TUITION: $22,433

OUT-OF-STATE TUITION: $34,785

TYPE OF SCHOOL: Public

UNIVERSITY OF MINNESOTA—DULUTH

Medical School
180 Medicine
1035 University Drive
Duluth, MN 55812
Phone: 218-726-8511
Fax: 218-726-7057
medadmis@d.umn.edu

www.med.umn.edu/duluth

TOTAL ENROLLMENT: 106

% ACCEPTED: 7.90%

% MALE/FEMALE RATIO: 50/50

% UNDERREP. MINORITIES: 6%

APPLICATION DEADLINE: 11/15

APPLICATION NOTIFICATION: Rolling

EARLY APPLICATION DEADLINE: 8/1

EARLY APPLICATION NOTIFICATION: 10/1

TRANSFERS ACCEPTED: No

ADMISSIONS DEFFERABLE: Yes

APPLICATION FEE: $75

INTERVIEW TIMEFRAMES: October-April

MCAT SCORES: 27.92

GPA: 3.59

IN-STATE TUITION: $44,890

OUT-OF-STATE TUITION: $51,785

TYPE OF SCHOOL: Public

UNIVERSITY OF MINNESOTA— TWIN CITIES

Medical School
Office of Admissions
P.O. Box 293
420 Delaware Street, Southeast
Minneapolis, MN 55455
Phone: 612-624-1188
Fax: 612-625-8228
meded@umn.edu
www.medn.umn.edu

TOTAL ENROLLMENT: 910

% ACCEPTED: 11.40%

% MALE/FEMALE RATIO: NA

% UNDERREP. MINORITIES: NA

APPLICATION DEADLINE: 11/15

APPLICATION NOTIFICATION: Rolling

EARLY APPLICATION DEADLINE: 6/1-8/1

EARLY APPLICATION NOTIFICATION: 10/1

TRANSFERS ACCEPTED: Yes

ADMISSIONS DEFFERABLE: Yes

APPLICATION FEE: $75

INTERVIEW TIMEFRAMES: September-March

MCAT SCORES: 31.5

GPA: 3.68

IN-STATE TUITION: $37,077

OUT-OF-STATE TUITION: $43,397

TYPE OF SCHOOL: Public

UNIVERSITY OF MISSISSIPPI

Medical Center
2500 North State Street
Jackson, MS 39216
Phone: 601-984-5010
Fax: 601-984-5008
admitmd.som.umsmed.edu
www.som.umc.edu

TOTAL ENROLLMENT: 519

% ACCEPTED: 50.00%

% MALE/FEMALE RATIO: 59/41

% UNDERREP. MINORITIES: 14%

APPLICATION DEADLINE: 10/15

APPLICATION NOTIFICATION: 3/15

EARLY APPLICATION DEADLINE: 8/1

EARLY APPLICATION NOTIFICATION: 10/1

TRANSFERS ACCEPTED: Yes

ADMISSIONS DEFFERABLE: Yes

APPLICATION FEE: NA

INTERVIEW TIMEFRAMES: August-January

MCAT SCORES: 28.28

GPA: 3.7

IN-STATE TUITION: $22,649

OUT-OF-STATE TUITION: $29,327

TYPE OF SCHOOL: Public

UNIVERSITY OF MISSOURI—COLUMBIA

School of Medicine
Ma215 Medical Sciences Building
Columiba, MO 65212
Phone: 573-882-9219
Fax: 573-884-2988
nolkej@health.missouri.edu
www.muhealth.org/~medicine

TOTAL ENROLLMENT: 375

% ACCEPTED: 16.20%

% MALE/FEMALE RATIO: 51/49

% UNDERREP. MINORITIES: 7%

APPLICATION DEADLINE: 11/1

APPLICATION NOTIFICATION: 3/15

EARLY APPLICATION DEADLINE: 8/1

EARLY APPLICATION NOTIFICATION: 10/1

TRANSFERS ACCEPTED: Yes

ADMISSIONS DEFFERABLE: Yes

APPLICATION FEE: $75

INTERVIEW TIMEFRAMES: October-April

MCAT SCORES: 29.85

GPA: 3.75

IN-STATE TUITION: $32,554

OUT-OF-STATE TUITION: $54,279

TYPE OF SCHOOL: Public

UNIVERSITY OF MISSOURI— KANSAS CITY

School of Medicine
Council on Selection
2411 Holmes
Kansas City, MO 64108-2792
Phone: 816-235-1870
Fax: 816-235-6579
morgeneggm@umkc.edu
www.umkc.edu/med

TOTAL ENROLLMENT: 630

% ACCEPTED: 37.00%

% MALE/FEMALE RATIO: 40/60

% UNDERREP. MINORITIES: 9%

APPLICATION DEADLINE: 11/15

APPLICATION NOTIFICATION: 4/1

EARLY APPLICATION DEADLINE: NA

EARLY APPLICATION NOTIFICATION: NA

TRANSFERS ACCEPTED: No

ADMISSIONS DEFFERABLE: No

APPLICATION FEE: $35/$50

INTERVIEW TIMEFRAMES: December-March

MCAT SCORES: NA

GPA: NA

IN-STATE TUITION: $36,292

OUT-OF-STATE TUITION: $61,588

TYPE OF SCHOOL: Public

UNIVERSITY OF MONTREAL

Faculté De Medécine
CP 6128
Succursale Centre-ville
Montreal, QC H3C 3J7
Phone: 514-343-6265
Fax: NA
facmed@meddir.umontreal.ca
www.med.umontreal.ca

TOTAL ENROLLMENT: NA

% ACCEPTED: NA

% MALE/FEMALE RATIO: NA

% UNDERREP. MINORITIES: NA

APPLICATION DEADLINE: 3/1

APPLICATION NOTIFICATION: 3/31

EARLY APPLICATION DEADLINE: NA

EARLY APPLICATION NOTIFICATION: NA

TRANSFERS ACCEPTED: NA

ADMISSIONS DEFFERABLE: No

APPLICATION FEE: $45

INTERVIEW TIMEFRAMES: NA

MCAT SCORES: NA

GPA: NA

IN-STATE TUITION: $2,605

OUT-OF-STATE TUITION: $12,866

TYPE OF SCHOOL: Public

UNIVERSITY OF NEBRASKA MEDICAL CENTER

College of Medicine
986585 Nebraska Medical Center
Omaha, NE 68198-6585
Phone: 402-559-6140
Fax: 402-559-6840
grrogers@unmc.edu
www.unmc.edu/uncom

TOTAL ENROLLMENT: 475

% ACCEPTED: 15.60%

% MALE/FEMALE RATIO: 59/41

% UNDERREP. MINORITIES: 10%

APPLICATION DEADLINE: 11/1

APPLICATION NOTIFICATION: Rolling

EARLY APPLICATION DEADLINE: 8/1

EARLY APPLICATION NOTIFICATION: 10/1

TRANSFERS ACCEPTED: Yes

ADMISSIONS DEFFERABLE: No

APPLICATION FEE: $45

INTERVIEW TIMEFRAMES: October-February

MCAT SCORES: 29.1

GPA: 3.75

IN-STATE TUITION: $36,775

OUT-OF-STATE TUITION: $64,405

TYPE OF SCHOOL: Public

UNIVERSITY OF NEVADA

School of Medicine
Office of Admissions
Reno, NV 89557
Phone: 702-784-6063
Fax: 702-784-6194
asa@scs.unr.edu

www.unr.edu.unr/med/html

TOTAL ENROLLMENT: 208

% ACCEPTED: 6.00%

% MALE/FEMALE RATIO: 61/39

% UNDERREP. MINORITIES: 5%

APPLICATION DEADLINE: 11/1

APPLICATION NOTIFICATION: NA

EARLY APPLICATION DEADLINE: 6/1-8/1

EARLY APPLICATION NOTIFICATION: 10/1

TRANSFERS ACCEPTED: Yes

ADMISSIONS DEFFERABLE: Yes

APPLICATION FEE: $45

INTERVIEW TIMEFRAMES: September-January

MCAT SCORES: NA

GPA: 3.6

IN-STATE TUITION: $11,607

OUT-OF-STATE TUITION: $29,185

TYPE OF SCHOOL: Public

UNVERSITY OF NEW MEXICO

School of Medicine
MSC 08 4690
BMSB Room 106
Albuquerque, NM 87131
Phone: 505-272-4766
Fax: 505-272-8239
somadmissions@salud.unm.edu

www.hsc.edu/som/

TOTAL ENROLLMENT: 324

% ACCEPTED: 9.30%

% MALE/FEMALE RATIO: 43/57

% UNDERREP. MINORITIES: 43%

APPLICATION DEADLINE: 11/15

APPLICATION NOTIFICATION: 3/15

EARLY APPLICATION DEADLINE: 8/1

EARLY APPLICATION NOTIFICATION: 10/1

TRANSFERS ACCEPTED: Yes

ADMISSIONS DEFFERABLE: Yes

APPLICATION FEE: $50

INTERVIEW TIMEFRAMES: June-March

MCAT SCORES: 28.4

GPA: 3.59

IN-STATE TUITION: $26,164

OUT-OF-STATE TUITION: $50,303

TYPE OF SCHOOL: Public

UNIVERSITY OF NORTH CAROLINA

School of Medicine at Chapel Hill
UNC School of Medicine
121 Macnider Building, CB #9500
Chapel Hill, NC 27599
Phone: 919-962-8331
Fax: 919-966-9930
admissions@med.unc.edu

www.med.unc.edu

TOTAL ENROLLMENT: NA

% ACCEPTED: NA

% MALE/FEMALE RATIO: NA

% UNDERREP. MINORITIES: NA

APPLICATION DEADLINE: NA

APPLICATION NOTIFICATION: NA

EARLY APPLICATION DEADLINE: NA

EARLY APPLICATION NOTIFICATION: NA

TRANSFERS ACCEPTED: NA

ADMISSIONS DEFFERABLE: NA

APPLICATION FEE: NA

INTERVIEW TIMEFRAMES: August-March

MCAT SCORES: 31.3

GPA: 3.7

IN-STATE TUITION: $21,366

OUT-OF-STATE TUITION: $46,834

TYPE OF SCHOOL: Public

UNVERSITY OF NORTH DAKOTA

School of Medicine and Health Sciences
501 North Columbia Road
P.O. Box 9037
Grand Forks, ND 58202-9037
Phone: 701-777-4221
Fax: 701-777-4342
jdheit@medicine.nodak.edu

www.med.und.nodak.edu

TOTAL ENROLLMENT: 236

% ACCEPTED: 33.60%

% MALE/FEMALE RATIO: 48/52

% UNDERREP. MINORITIES: 12%

APPLICATION DEADLINE: 11/1

APPLICATION NOTIFICATION: 1/15

EARLY APPLICATION DEADLINE: NA

EARLY APPLICATION NOTIFICATION: NA

TRANSFERS ACCEPTED: No

ADMISSIONS DEFFERABLE: Yes

APPLICATION FEE: $50

INTERVIEW TIMEFRAMES: December-January

MCAT SCORES: 27.4

GPA: 3.7

IN-STATE TUITION: $31,124

OUT-OF-STATE TUITION: $62,698

TYPE OF SCHOOL: Public

UNIVERSITY OF OKLAHOMA

College of Medicine
P.O. Box 26901
Oklahoma City, OK 73190
Phone: 405-271-2331
Fax: 405-271-3032
adminmed@ouhsc.edu
www.medicine.ouhsc.edu

TOTAL ENROLLMENT: 575

% ACCEPTED: 19.60%

% MALE/FEMALE RATIO: 61/39

% UNDERREP. MINORITIES: 27%

APPLICATION DEADLINE: 10/15

APPLICATION NOTIFICATION: NA

EARLY APPLICATION DEADLINE: NA

EARLY APPLICATION NOTIFICATION: NA

TRANSFERS ACCEPTED: Yes

ADMISSIONS DEFFERABLE: No

APPLICATION FEE: $65

INTERVIEW TIMEFRAMES: September-February

MCAT SCORES: 28.93

GPA: 3.68

IN-STATE TUITION: $22,640

OUT-OF-STATE TUITION: $44,728

TYPE OF SCHOOL: Public

UNIVERSITY OF OTTOWA

451 Smyth Road, Room 2046
Ottawa, ON K1H 8M5
Phone: 613-562-5409
Fax: 613-562-5651
admissmd@uottawa.ca
www.medicine.uottowa.ca/eng/
  undergraduate.html

TOTAL ENROLLMENT: NA

% ACCEPTED: 7.83%

% MALE/FEMALE RATIO: NA

% UNDERREP. MINORITIES: NA

APPLICATION DEADLINE: 10/15

APPLICATION NOTIFICATION: 5/31

EARLY APPLICATION DEADLINE: NA

EARLY APPLICATION NOTIFICATION: NA

TRANSFERS ACCEPTED: Yes

ADMISSIONS DEFFERABLE: Yes

APPLICATION FEE: $175

INTERVIEW TIMEFRAMES: NA

MCAT SCORES: NA

GPA: 3.65

IN-STATE TUITION: $14,552

OUT-OF-STATE TUITION: Na

TYPE OF SCHOOL: Public

University of Pennsylvania

School of Medicine
Director of Admissions
Edward J. Stemmler Hall, Suite 100
Philadelphia, PA 19104
Phone: 215-898-8001
Fax: 215-573-6645
admiss@mail.med.upenn.edu
www.med.upenn.edu

Total Enrollment: 720

% Accepted: 2.63%

% Male/Female Ratio: 51/49

% Underrep. Minorities: 17%

Application Deadline: 10/15

Application Notification: 3/15

Early Application Deadline: NA

Early Application Notification: NA

Transfers Accepted: No

Admissions Defferable: Yes

Application Fee: $80

Interview Timeframes: October-February

MCAT Scores: NA

GPA: NA

In-state Tuition: $54,888

Out-of-state Tuition: $54,888

Type of School: Private

University of Pittsburgh

School of Medicine
Office of Admissions
518 Scaife Hall
Pittsburgh, PA 15261
Phone: 412-648-9891
Fax: 412-648-8768
admissions@medschool.pitt.edu
www.medschool.pitt.edu

Total Enrollment: 592

% Accepted: NA

% Male/Female Ratio: 52/48

% Underrep. Minorities: 9%

Application Deadline: 12/1

Application Notification: 10/15

Early Application Deadline: 6/1-8/1

Early Application Notification: 10/1

Transfers Accepted: Yes

Admissions Defferable: Yes

Application Fee: $75

Interview Timeframes: September-April

MCAT Scores: NA

GPA: NA

In-state Tuition: $32,684

Out-of-state Tuition: $38,476

Type of School: Public

UNIVERSITY OF PUERTO RICO

Medical Sciences Campus
A-878 Main Building
P.O. Box 365067
San Juan, PR 00936-5067
Phone: 787-758-2525 Ext. 1800
Fax: 787-756-8475
marrivera@rcm.upr.edu

www.rcm.upr.edu

TOTAL ENROLLMENT: 1716

% ACCEPTED: NA

% MALE/FEMALE RATIO: NA

% UNDERREP. MINORITIES: NA

APPLICATION DEADLINE: 12/1

APPLICATION NOTIFICATION: Rolling

EARLY APPLICATION DEADLINE: 6/1

EARLY APPLICATION NOTIFICATION: Rolling

TRANSFERS ACCEPTED: NA

ADMISSIONS DEFFERABLE: NA

APPLICATION FEE: $15

INTERVIEW TIMEFRAMES: NA

MCAT SCORES: NA

GPA: NA

IN-STATE TUITION: $18,603

OUT-OF-STATE TUITION: NA

TYPE OF SCHOOL: Public

UNIVERSITY OF ROCHESTER

School of Medicine and Dentistry
Medical Center
P.O. Box 601A
Rochester, NY 14642
Phone: 585-275-4539
Fax: 585-756-5479
mdadmish@urmc.rochester.edu

www.urmc.rochester.edu/smd/admiss

TOTAL ENROLLMENT: 433

% ACCEPTED: 7.44%

% MALE/FEMALE RATIO: 45/55

% UNDERREP. MINORITIES: 14%

APPLICATION DEADLINE: 10/15

APPLICATION NOTIFICATION: 11/1

EARLY APPLICATION DEADLINE: NA

EARLY APPLICATION NOTIFICATION: NA

TRANSFERS ACCEPTED: No

ADMISSIONS DEFFERABLE: Yes

APPLICATION FEE: $75

INTERVIEW TIMEFRAMES: September-February

MCAT SCORES: 32.3

GPA: 3.68

IN-STATE TUITION: $49,185

OUT-OF-STATE TUITION: $49,185

TYPE OF SCHOOL: Private

UNIVERSITY OF SASKATCHEWAN

College of Medicine
A204 Health Science Building
107 Wiggins Road
Saskatoon, SK Canada
Phone: 306-966-8554
Fax: 306-966-2601
med.admissions@usask.ca
www.usask.ca/medicine

TOTAL ENROLLMENT: 60

% ACCEPTED: 13.00%

% MALE/FEMALE RATIO: 52/48

% UNDERREP. MINORITIES: 5%

APPLICATION DEADLINE: 12/1

APPLICATION NOTIFICATION: 5/16

EARLY APPLICATION DEADLINE: NA

EARLY APPLICATION NOTIFICATION: NA

TRANSFERS ACCEPTED: No

ADMISSIONS DEFFERABLE: Yes

APPLICATION FEE: $40

INTERVIEW TIMEFRAMES: March

MCAT SCORES: 28.9

GPA: NA

IN-STATE TUITION: $17,922

OUT-OF-STATE TUITION: $17,922

TYPE OF SCHOOL: Public

UNIVERSITY OF SHERBROOKE

2500 Boulevard De L'université
Sherbrooke, QC J1K 2R1
Phone: 819-821-7686
Fax: NA
stic-med@usherbrooke.ca
www.usherbrooke.ca/medicine

TOTAL ENROLLMENT: NA

% ACCEPTED: NA

% MALE/FEMALE RATIO: NA

% UNDERREP. MINORITIES: NA

APPLICATION DEADLINE: 3/1

APPLICATION NOTIFICATION: Rolling

EARLY APPLICATION DEADLINE: NA

EARLY APPLICATION NOTIFICATION: NA

TRANSFERS ACCEPTED: NA

ADMISSIONS DEFFERABLE: No

APPLICATION FEE: $30

INTERVIEW TIMEFRAMES: NA

MCAT SCORES: NA

GPA: NA

IN-STATE TUITION: $3,127

OUT-OF-STATE TUITION: $15,127

TYPE OF SCHOOL: Public

UNIVERSITY OF SOUTH ALABAMA

College of Medicine
Office of Admissions, 241 CSAB
Mobile, AL 36688
Phone: 251-460-7176
Fax: 251-460-6278
mscott@usouthal.edu

www.usouthal.edu/usa/deps-grd.html

TOTAL ENROLLMENT: 280

% ACCEPTED: 14.34%

% MALE/FEMALE RATIO: 49/51

% UNDERREP. MINORITIES: 11%

APPLICATION DEADLINE: 11/15

APPLICATION NOTIFICATION: Rolling

EARLY APPLICATION DEADLINE: 6/1-8/1

EARLY APPLICATION NOTIFICATION: 10/1

TRANSFERS ACCEPTED: Yes

ADMISSIONS DEFFERABLE: Yes

APPLICATION FEE: $75

INTERVIEW TIMEFRAMES: September-March

MCAT SCORES: 31

GPA: 3.7

IN-STATE TUITION: $19,605

OUT-OF-STATE TUITION: $30,645

TYPE OF SCHOOL: Public

UNIVERSITY OF SOUTH CAROLINA

School of Medicine
Admissions Office
Columbia, SC 29208
Phone: 803-733-3325
Fax: 803-733-3328
mills@gw.med.sc.edu

www.med.sc.edu

TOTAL ENROLLMENT: 297

% ACCEPTED: 12.70%

% MALE/FEMALE RATIO: 53/47

% UNDERREP. MINORITIES: 20%

APPLICATION DEADLINE: 12/1

APPLICATION NOTIFICATION: 10/15

EARLY APPLICATION DEADLINE: 6/1-8/1

EARLY APPLICATION NOTIFICATION: 10/1

TRANSFERS ACCEPTED: Yes

ADMISSIONS DEFFERABLE: Yes

APPLICATION FEE: $45

INTERVIEW TIMEFRAMES: August-April

MCAT SCORES: 26

GPA: 3.5

IN-STATE TUITION: $34,000

OUT-OF-STATE TUITION: $65,970

TYPE OF SCHOOL: Public

The University of South Dakota

Sanford School of Medicine
Office of Medical Student Affairs
414 East Clark Street
Vermillion, SD 57069
Phone: 605-677-6886
Fax: 605-677-5109
usdsmsa@.usd.edu
www.usd.edu/med/md

Total Enrollment: 206

% Accepted: 9.21%

% Male/Female Ratio: 52/48

% Underrep. Minorities: 5%

Application Deadline: 11/15

Application Notification: Rolling

Early Application Deadline: NA

Early Application Notification: NA

Transfers Accepted: Yes

Admissions Defferable: Yes

Application Fee: $35

Interview Timeframes: October-February

MCAT Scores: 28.06

GPA: 3.66

In-state Tuition: $36,106

Out-of-state Tuition: $54,572

Type of School: Public

University of South Florida

College of Medicine
12901 Bruce B. Downs Boulevard, MDC-3
Tampa, FL 33612
Phone: 813-974-2229
Fax: 813-974-4990
md-admissions@lyris.hsc.usf.edu
www.hsc.usf.edu/medicine/mdadmissions

Total Enrollment: 458

% Accepted: 6.40%

% Male/Female Ratio: 47/53

% Underrep. Minorities: 37%

Application Deadline: 12/1

Application Notification: 10/15

Early Application Deadline: 8/15

Early Application Notification: 10/1

Transfers Accepted: Yes

Admissions Defferable: Yes

Application Fee: $30

Interview Timeframes: September-April

MCAT Scores: 29

GPA: 3.68

In-state Tuition: $29,814

Out-of-state Tuition: $61,848

Type of School: Public

UNIVERSITY OF SOUTHERN CALIFORNIA

Keck School of Medicine
1975 Zonal Avenue, Kam 100-C
Los Angeles, CA 90089-9021
Phone: 323-442-2552
Fax: 323-441-2433
medadmit@hsc.usc.edu
www.usc.edu/medicine

TOTAL ENROLLMENT: 659

% ACCEPTED: 6.13%

% MALE/FEMALE RATIO: 52/48

% UNDERREP. MINORITIES: 17%

APPLICATION DEADLINE: 10/1

APPLICATION NOTIFICATION: 4/2

EARLY APPLICATION DEADLINE: 8/1

EARLY APPLICATION NOTIFICATION: 10/1

TRANSFERS ACCEPTED: Yes

ADMISSIONS DEFFERABLE: Yes

APPLICATION FEE: $90

INTERVIEW TIMEFRAMES: NA

MCAT SCORES: 30.7

GPA: 3.6

IN-STATE TUITION: $48,067

OUT-OF-STATE TUITION: $48,067

TYPE OF SCHOOL: Private

UNIVERSITY OF TENNESSEE—MEMPHIS

College of Medicine
Admissions Office
790 Madison Avenue, Room 307
Memphis, TN 38163
Phone: 901-448-5559
Fax: 901-448-1740
www.utmem.edu/medicine

TOTAL ENROLLMENT: 686

% ACCEPTED: NA

% MALE/FEMALE RATIO: 61/39

% UNDERREP. MINORITIES: 15%

APPLICATION DEADLINE: 11/15

APPLICATION NOTIFICATION: 10/15-4/1

EARLY APPLICATION DEADLINE: NA

EARLY APPLICATION NOTIFICATION: NA

TRANSFERS ACCEPTED: Yes

ADMISSIONS DEFFERABLE: Yes

APPLICATION FEE: $50

INTERVIEW TIMEFRAMES: October-March

MCAT SCORES: NA

GPA: NA

IN-STATE TUITION: $12,469

OUT-OF-STATE TUITION: $21,133

TYPE OF SCHOOL: Public

University of Texas

Medical Branch at Galveston
School of Medicine
Office of Admissions, G-210
Ashbel Smith Building
Galveston, TX 77555-1317
Phone: 409-772-3517
Fax: 409-772-5733
pwylie@mspo4.med.edu
www.utmb.edu

Total Enrollment: 821

% Accepted: 1.33%

% Male/Female Ratio: 59/41

% Underrep. Minorities: 15%

Application Deadline: 10/15

Application Notification: 1/15

Early Application Deadline: NA

Early Application Notification: NA

Transfers Accepted: No

Admissions Defferable: Yes

Application Fee: $45

Interview Timeframes: November-December

MCAT Scores: NA

GPA: NA

In-state Tuition: $4,000

Out-of-state Tuition: $4,000

Type of School: Public

University of Texas Health Science Center at Houston

Medical School at Houston
Office of Admissions, MSB G420
Houston, TX 77030
Phone: 713-500-5116
Fax: 713-500-0604
msadmissions@uth.tmc.edu
www.med.uth.tmc.edu

Total Enrollment: 848

% Accepted: 7.90%

% Male/Female Ratio: 52/48

% Underrep. Minorities: 27%

Application Deadline: 10/15

Application Notification: 2/1

Early Application Deadline: NA

Early Application Notification: NA

Transfers Accepted: No

Admissions Defferable: No

Application Fee: $55

Interview Timeframes: August-January

MCAT Scores: 28.6

GPA: 3.66

In-state Tuition: $25,165

Out-of-state Tuition: $39,118

Type of School: Public

UNIVERSITY OF TEXAS HEALTH SCIENCE CENTER AT SAN ANTONIO

Medical School at San Antonio
Medical School Admissions Office
7703 FLoyd Curl Drive
San Antonio, TX 78229
Phone: 210-567-2665
Fax: 210-568-2685
chapab@uthscsa.edu
www.uthscsa.edu

TOTAL ENROLLMENT: 814

% ACCEPTED: NA

% MALE/FEMALE RATIO: 58/48

% UNDERREP. MINORITIES: 16%

APPLICATION DEADLINE: 10/1

APPLICATION NOTIFICATION: 1/15

EARLY APPLICATION DEADLINE: NA

EARLY APPLICATION NOTIFICATION: NA

TRANSFERS ACCEPTED: Yes

ADMISSIONS DEFFERABLE: No

APPLICATION FEE: $45

INTERVIEW TIMEFRAMES: August-December

MCAT SCORES: NA

GPA: NA

IN-STATE TUITION: NA

OUT-OF-STATE TUITION: NA

TYPE OF SCHOOL: Public

UNIVERSITY OF TEXAS SOUTHWESTERN

Medical School at Dallas
5323 Harry Hines Boulevard
Dallas, TX 75390-9162
Phone: 214-648-5617
Fax: 214-648-3289
admissions@utsouthwestern.edu
www.utsouthwestern.edu

TOTAL ENROLLMENT: 904

% ACCEPTED: 13.30%

% MALE/FEMALE RATIO: 56/44

% UNDERREP. MINORITIES: 20%

APPLICATION DEADLINE: 10/15

APPLICATION NOTIFICATION: 11/15

EARLY APPLICATION DEADLINE: NA

EARLY APPLICATION NOTIFICATION: NA

TRANSFERS ACCEPTED: Yes

ADMISSIONS DEFFERABLE: Yes

APPLICATION FEE: $65

INTERVIEW TIMEFRAMES: August-December

MCAT SCORES: 33

GPA: 3.78

IN-STATE TUITION: $3,247

OUT-OF-STATE TUITION: $25,672

TYPE OF SCHOOL: Public

University of Toronto

Faculy of Medicine
315 Bloor Street
West Toronto, ON M5S 1A3
Phone: 416-978-2190
Fax: 416-978-7022

www.utoronto.ca

Total Enrollment: NA

% Accepted: NA

% Male/Female Ratio: NA

% Underrep. Minorities: NA

Application Deadline: 10/15

Application Notification: 5/31

Early Application Deadline: NA

Early Application Notification: NA

Transfers Accepted: No

Admissions Defferable: Yes

Application Fee: $75

Interview Timeframes: NA

MCAT Scores: NA

GPA: NA

In-state Tuition: $14,919

Out-of-state Tuition: $25,248

Type of School: Public

University of Utah

School of Medicine
Office of Admissions, 30 North
1900 East #1C029
Salt Lake City, UT 84132-2101
Phone: 801-581-7498
Fax: 801-581-2931
Deans.admissions@hsc.utah.edu

Http://uuhsc.utah.edu/som

Total Enrollment: 409

% Accepted: 9.60%

% Male/Female Ratio: 63/37

% Underrep. Minorities: 12%

Application Deadline: 11/1

Application Notification: NA

Early Application Deadline: NA

Early Application Notification: NA

Transfers Accepted: Yes

Admissions Defferable: Yes

Application Fee: $100

Interview Timeframes: September-February

MCAT Scores: 28

GPA: 3.6

In-state Tuition: $18,320

Out-of-state Tuition: $33,479

Type of School: Public

UNIVERSITY OF VERMONT

College of Medicine
89 Beaumont Avenue
E215 Given Building
Burlington, VT 05405
Phone: 802-656-2154
Fax: 802-656-9663
medadmissions@uvm.edu
www.med.uvm.edu

TOTAL ENROLLMENT: 400

% ACCEPTED: 4.00%

% MALE/FEMALE RATIO: 41/59

% UNDERREP. MINORITIES: 20%

APPLICATION DEADLINE: 11/1

APPLICATION NOTIFICATION: 10/15

EARLY APPLICATION DEADLINE: 8/1

EARLY APPLICATION NOTIFICATION: 10/1

TRANSFERS ACCEPTED: Yes

ADMISSIONS DEFFERABLE: Yes

APPLICATION FEE: $85

INTERVIEW TIMEFRAMES: September-March

MCAT SCORES: 28.2

GPA: 3.5

IN-STATE TUITION: $41,759

OUT-OF-STATE TUITION: $59,069

TYPE OF SCHOOL: Public

UNIVERSITY OF VIRGINIA

School of Medicine
P.O. Box 800725
Charlottesville, VA 22908
Phone: 804-924-5571
Fax: 804-982-2586
bab7g@virginia.edu
www.med.virginia.edu/home.html

TOTAL ENROLLMENT: 556

% ACCEPTED: 3.91%

% MALE/FEMALE RATIO: 50/50

% UNDERREP. MINORITIES: 8%

APPLICATION DEADLINE: 11/1

APPLICATION NOTIFICATION: 10/15

EARLY APPLICATION DEADLINE: NA

EARLY APPLICATION NOTIFICATION: NA

TRANSFERS ACCEPTED: Yes

ADMISSIONS DEFFERABLE: Yes

APPLICATION FEE: $75

INTERVIEW TIMEFRAMES: NA

MCAT SCORES: 32.23

GPA: 3.74

IN-STATE TUITION: $41,700

OUT-OF-STATE TUITION: $51,700

TYPE OF SCHOOL: Public

University of Washington

School of Medicine
Admissions Office
A-300 Health Sciences
P.O. Box 356340
Seattle, Wa 98195
Phone: 206-543-7212
Fax: 206-616-3341
askuwsom@u.washington.edu
www.washington.edu/medicine/som

Total Enrollment: 734

% Accepted: 7.33%

% Male/Female Ratio: 52/48

% Underrep. Minorities: 10%

Application Deadline: 11/1

Application Notification: 11/1

Early Application Deadline: NA

Early Application Notification: NA

Transfers Accepted: Yes

Admissions Defferable: Yes

Application Fee: $35

Interview Timeframes: October-April

MCAT Scores: 32.2

GPA: 3.7

In-state Tuition: $12,450

Out-of-state Tuition: $29,391

Type of School: Public

University of Western Ontario

Admission and Student Affairs
Health Sciences Building
London, Ontario N6A 5C1
Phone: 519-661-3744
Fax: 519-661-3797
admissions@schulich.uwo.ca
www.schulich.uwo.ca

Total Enrollment: 534

% Accepted: 7.10%

% Male/Female Ratio: 55/45

% Underrep. Minorities: NA

Application Deadline: 10/15

Application Notification: 5/15

Early Application Deadline: NA

Early Application Notification: NA

Transfers Accepted: No

Admissions Defferable: No

Application Fee: $175

Interview Timeframes: NA

MCAT Scores: 29

GPA: 3.7

In-state Tuition: $30,629

Out-of-state Tuition: $30,629

Type of School: Public

UNIVERSITY OF WISCONSIN—MADISON

School of Medicine and Public Health
2130 Health Sciences Learning Center
750 Highland Avenue
Madison, WI 53705
Phone: 608-263-4925
Fax: 608-262-4226
lwall@wisc.edu

www.med.wisc.edu

TOTAL ENROLLMENT: 607

% ACCEPTED: 29.63%

% MALE/FEMALE RATIO: 48/52

% UNDERREP. MINORITIES: 8%

APPLICATION DEADLINE: 11/1

APPLICATION NOTIFICATION: Rolling

EARLY APPLICATION DEADLINE: 8/1 and 9/1

EARLY APPLICATION NOTIFICATION: 10/1

TRANSFERS ACCEPTED: Yes

ADMISSIONS DEFFERABLE: Yes

APPLICATION FEE: $45

INTERVIEW TIMEFRAMES: August-March

MCAT SCORES: 31.2

GPA: 3.7

IN-STATE TUITION: $34,882

OUT-OF-STATE TUITION: $46,006

TYPE OF SCHOOL: Public

VANDERBILT UNIVERSITY

School of Medicine
215 Light Hall
Nashiville, TN 37232-0685
Phone: 615-322-2145
Fax: 615-343-8397
hal.helderman@vanderbilt.edu

www.mc.vanderbilt.edu/medschool/
   admissions.index.php

TOTAL ENROLLMENT: 432

% ACCEPTED: 6.70%

% MALE/FEMALE RATIO: 53/47

% UNDERREP. MINORITIES: 9%

APPLICATION DEADLINE: 11/15

APPLICATION NOTIFICATION: Rolling

EARLY APPLICATION DEADLINE: 6/1-8/1

EARLY APPLICATION NOTIFICATION: 10/1

TRANSFERS ACCEPTED: Yes

ADMISSIONS DEFFERABLE: Yes

APPLICATION FEE: $50

INTERVIEW TIMEFRAMES: September-March

MCAT SCORES: 33.81

GPA: 3.73

IN-STATE TUITION: $49,620

OUT-OF-STATE TUITION: $49,620

TYPE OF SCHOOL: Private

Virginia Commonwealth University

School of Medicine
P.O. Box 980565
Richmond, VA
Phone: 804-828-9629
Fax: 804-828-1246
somume@hsc.vcu.edu

www.medschool.vcu.edu

Total Enrollment: 698

% Accepted: 11.40%

% Male/Female Ratio: 51/49

% Underrep. Minorities: 7%

Application Deadline: 11/15

Application Notification: 10/15

Early Application Deadline: 6/1-8/1

Early Application Notification: 10/1

Transfers Accepted: Yes

Admissions Defferable: Yes

Application Fee: $80

Interview Timeframes: August-March

MCAT Scores: 28.8

GPA: 3.5

In-state Tuition: $23,441

Out-of-state Tuition: $41,766

Type of School: Public

Wake Forest University

School of Medicine
Office of Admissions
Medical Center Boulevard
Winston-salem, NC 27157-1090
Phone: 336-716-4264
Fax: 910-716-9593
medadmit@wfubmc.edu

www.wfubmc.edu

Total Enrollment: 431

% Accepted: 4.70%

% Male/Female Ratio: 56/44

% Underrep. Minorities: 30%

Application Deadline: 11/1

Application Notification: Rolling

Early Application Deadline: 6/1-8/1

Early Application Notification: 10/1

Transfers Accepted: Yes

Admissions Defferable: Yes

Application Fee: $55

Interview Timeframes: September-March

MCAT Scores: 30.3

GPA: 3.63

In-state Tuition: $50,942

Out-of-state Tuition: $50,942

Type of School: Private

WASHINGTON UNIVERSITY IN ST. LOUIS

School of Medicine
Office of Admissions
Box 8107
660 South Euclid Street
St. Louis, MO 63110
Phone: 314-362-6848
Fax: 314-362-4658
wumscoa@msnotes.wustl.edu

www.medschool.wustl.edu/admissions

TOTAL ENROLLMENT: 578

% ACCEPTED: 9.00%

% MALE/FEMALE RATIO: 55/45

% UNDERREP. MINORITIES: 40%

APPLICATION DEADLINE: 12/1

APPLICATION NOTIFICATION: Rolling

EARLY APPLICATION DEADLINE: NA

EARLY APPLICATION NOTIFICATION: NA

TRANSFERS ACCEPTED: Yes

ADMISSIONS DEFFERABLE: Yes

APPLICATION FEE: $50

INTERVIEW TIMEFRAMES: September-March

MCAT SCORES: 36.4

GPA: 3.8

IN-STATE TUITION: $38,645

OUT-OF-STATE TUITION: $38,645

TYPE OF SCHOOL: Private

WAYNE STATE UNIVERSITY

School of Medicine
Admissions
540 East Canfield, Suite 1310
Detroit, MI 48201
Phone: 313-577-1466
Fax: 313-577-9420
admissions@med.wayne.edu

www.med.wayne.edu/admissions

TOTAL ENROLLMENT: NA

% ACCEPTED: 18.50%

% MALE/FEMALE RATIO: 100/0

% UNDERREP. MINORITIES: 12%

APPLICATION DEADLINE: 12/15

APPLICATION NOTIFICATION: 10/15

EARLY APPLICATION DEADLINE: 6/1-8/1

EARLY APPLICATION NOTIFICATION: 10/1

TRANSFERS ACCEPTED: Yes

ADMISSIONS DEFFERABLE: Yes

APPLICATION FEE: $50

INTERVIEW TIMEFRAMES: September-April

MCAT SCORES: 28.1

GPA: 3.5

IN-STATE TUITION: $15,204

OUT-OF-STATE TUITION: $30,556

TYPE OF SCHOOL: Public

WEST VIRGINIA UNIVERSITY

School of Medicine
Robert C. Byrd Health Sciences Center
P.O. Box 9111
Morgantown, WV 26506
Phone: 304-293-2408
Fax: 304-293-7814
medadmissions@hsc.wvu.edu
www.hsc.wvu.edu/som

TOTAL ENROLLMENT: 404

% ACCEPTED: 10.40%

% MALE/FEMALE RATIO: 60/40

% UNDERREP. MINORITIES: 2%

APPLICATION DEADLINE: 11/15

APPLICATION NOTIFICATION: Rolling

EARLY APPLICATION DEADLINE: 8/1

EARLY APPLICATION NOTIFICATION: 10/1

TRANSFERS ACCEPTED: Yes

ADMISSIONS DEFFERABLE: Yes

APPLICATION FEE: $100

INTERVIEW TIMEFRAMES: September-February

MCAT SCORES: 26.8

GPA: 3.66

IN-STATE TUITION: $30,300

OUT-OF-STATE TUITION: $50,702

TYPE OF SCHOOL: Public

WRIGHT STATE UNIVERSITY

Boonshoft School of Medicine
Office of Student Affairs/admissions
P.O. Box 1751
Dayton, OH 45401-1751
Phone: 937-775-2934
Fax: 937-775-3322
som_saa@desire.wright.edu
www.med.wright.edu

TOTAL ENROLLMENT: 375

% ACCEPTED: 8.30%

% MALE/FEMALE RATIO: 44/56

% UNDERREP. MINORITIES: 23%

APPLICATION DEADLINE: 11/15

APPLICATION NOTIFICATION: 10/15

EARLY APPLICATION DEADLINE: 8/1

EARLY APPLICATION NOTIFICATION: 10/1

TRANSFERS ACCEPTED: Yes

ADMISSIONS DEFFERABLE: Yes

APPLICATION FEE: $45

INTERVIEW TIMEFRAMES: September-March

MCAT SCORES: 30.58

GPA: 3.58

IN-STATE TUITION: $34,705

OUT-OF-STATE TUITION: $43,429

TYPE OF SCHOOL: Public

YALE UNIVERSITY

School of Medicine
Office of Admissions
367 Cedar Street
New Haven, CT 06510
Phone: 203-785-2643
Fax: 203-785-3234
medicalschool.admissions@
    quickmail.yale.edu

www.info.med.yale.edu/education/
admissions/index.html

TOTAL ENROLLMENT: 479

% ACCEPTED: NA

% MALE/FEMALE RATIO: 51/49

% UNDERREP. MINORITIES: 18%

APPLICATION DEADLINE: 10/15

APPLICATION NOTIFICATION: 3/15

EARLY APPLICATION DEADLINE: 6/1-8/1

EARLY APPLICATION NOTIFICATION: 10/1

TRANSFERS ACCEPTED: Yes

ADMISSIONS DEFFERABLE: Yes

APPLICATION FEE: $60

INTERVIEW TIMEFRAMES: October-February

MCAT SCORES: NA

GPA: NA

IN-STATE TUITION: $45,450

OUT-OF-STATE TUITION: $45,450

TYPE OF SCHOOL: Private

YESHIVA UNIVERSITY

Albert Einstein College of Medicine
1300 Morris Park Avenue
Bronx, NY 10461
Phone: 718-430-2106
Fax: 718-430-8825
admissions@aecom.yu.edu

www.aecom.yu.edu

TOTAL ENROLLMENT: 724

% ACCEPTED: 8.80%

% MALE/FEMALE RATIO: 51/49

% UNDERREP. MINORITIES: 7%

APPLICATION DEADLINE: 12/31

APPLICATION NOTIFICATION: 1/15

EARLY APPLICATION DEADLINE: 8/1

EARLY APPLICATION NOTIFICATION: 10/1

TRANSFERS ACCEPTED: No

ADMISSIONS DEFFERABLE: Yes

APPLICATION FEE: $90

INTERVIEW TIMEFRAMES: August-May

MCAT SCORES: 30.5

GPA: 3.6

IN-STATE TUITION: $43,125

OUT-OF-STATE TUITION: $43,125

TYPE OF SCHOOL: Private

NATUROPATHIC SCHOOLS

BASTYR UNIVERSITY

School of Naturopathic Medicine
14500 Juanita Drive Northeast
Kenmore, WA 98028
Phone: 425-602-3330
Fax: 425-602-3090
admissions@bastyr.edu
www.bastyr.edu

TOTAL ENROLLMENT: 477

% ACCEPTED: 75%

% MALE/FEMALE RATIO: 28/72

% UNDERREP. MINORITIES: 6%

APPLICATION DEADLINE: 2/1

APPLICATION NOTIFICATION: 4/15

EARLY APPLICATION DEADLINE: 11/

EARLY APPLICATION NOTIFICATION: 2/1

TRANSFERS ACCEPTED: Yes

ADMISSIONS DEFFERABLE: Yes

APPLICATION FEE: $75

INTERVIEW TIMEFRAMES: NA

MCAT SCORES: NA

GPA: 3.3

IN-STATE TUITION: $33,057

OUT-OF-STATE TUITION: $33,057

TYPE OF SCHOOL: Private

BOUCHER INSTITUTE OF NATUROPATHIC MEDICINE

300/435 Columbia Street
New Westminster, BC V3L 5N8
Phone: 604-777-9981
Fax: 604-777-9982
ssparlin@binm.org
www.binm.org

TOTAL ENROLLMENT: 80

% ACCEPTED: 50%

% MALE/FEMALE RATIO: NA

% UNDERREP. MINORITIES: NA

APPLICATION DEADLINE: 11/30

APPLICATION NOTIFICATION: NA

EARLY APPLICATION DEADLINE: NA

EARLY APPLICATION NOTIFICATION: NA

TRANSFERS ACCEPTED: Yes

ADMISSIONS DEFFERABLE: No

APPLICATION FEE: $100

INTERVIEW TIMEFRAMES: NA

MCAT SCORES: NA

GPA: NA

IN-STATE TUITION: $22,150

OUT-OF-STATE TUITION: $22,150

TYPE OF SCHOOL: Private

THE CANADIAN COLLEGE OF NATUROPATHIC MEDICINE

1255 Sheppard Avenue
Toronto, ON M2K 1E2
Phone: 416-498-1255 Ext. 245
Fax: 416-498-3197
info@ccnm.edu
www.ccnm.edu

TOTAL ENROLLMENT: 485

% ACCEPTED: NA

% MALE/FEMALE RATIO: 25/75

% UNDERREP. MINORITIES: NA

APPLICATION DEADLINE: NA

APPLICATION NOTIFICATION: NA

EARLY APPLICATION DEADLINE: NA

EARLY APPLICATION NOTIFICATION: NA

TRANSFERS ACCEPTED: Yes

ADMISSIONS DEFFERABLE: Yes

APPLICATION FEE: $150

INTERVIEW TIMEFRAMES: NA

MCAT SCORES: NA

GPA: 3.35

IN-STATE TUITION: $18,984

OUT-OF-STATE TUITION: $18,984

TYPE OF SCHOOL: Private

NATIONAL COLLEGE OF NATUROPATHIC MEDICINE

049 Southwest Porter Street
Portland, OR 97201
Phone: 503-552-1660
Fax: 503-499-0027
admissions@ncnm.edu
ncnm.edu

TOTAL ENROLLMENT: 351

% ACCEPTED: 84.60%

% MALE/FEMALE RATIO: 21/79

% UNDERREP. MINORITIES: 12%

APPLICATION DEADLINE: NA

APPLICATION NOTIFICATION: NA

EARLY APPLICATION DEADLINE: NA

EARLY APPLICATION NOTIFICATION: NA

TRANSFERS ACCEPTED: Yes

ADMISSIONS DEFFERABLE: Yes

APPLICATION FEE: $75

INTERVIEW TIMEFRAMES: NA

MCAT SCORES: NA

GPA: 3.36

IN-STATE TUITION: NA

OUT-OF-STATE TUITION: NA

TYPE OF SCHOOL: Private

SOUTHWEST COLLEGE OF NATUROPATHIC MEDICINE

2140 East Broadway Road
Tempe, AZ 85282
Phone: 888-882-7266
Fax: 480-858-9166
Admissions@scnm.edu
www.scnm.edu

TOTAL ENROLLMENT: 347

% ACCEPTED: 50.90%

% MALE/FEMALE RATIO: 31/69

% UNDERREP. MINORITIES: 35%

APPLICATION DEADLINE: NA

APPLICATION NOTIFICATION: NA

EARLY APPLICATION DEADLINE: NA

EARLY APPLICATION NOTIFICATION: NA

TRANSFERS ACCEPTED: Yes

ADMISSIONS DEFFERABLE: Yes

APPLICATION FEE: $65

INTERVIEW TIMEFRAMES: NA

MCAT SCORES: NA

GPA: 3.46

IN-STATE TUITION: $31,324

OUT-OF-STATE TUITION: $31,324

TYPE OF SCHOOL: Private

OSTEOPATHIC SCHOOLS

A.T. STILL UNIVERSITY OF HEALTH SCIENCES

Kirksville College of Osteopathic Medicine
800 West Jefferson
Kirksville, MO 63501
Phone: 660-626-2237
Fax: 660-626-2969
admissions@atsu.edu
www.atsu.edu

TOTAL ENROLLMENT: 670

% ACCEPTED: 14.70%

% MALE/FEMALE RATIO: 60/40

% UNDERREP. MINORITIES: 1%

APPLICATION DEADLINE: 2/1

APPLICATION NOTIFICATION: Rolling

EARLY APPLICATION DEADLINE: 8/1

EARLY APPLICATION NOTIFICATION: 10/15

TRANSFERS ACCEPTED: Yes

ADMISSIONS DEFFERABLE: Yes

APPLICATION FEE: $60

INTERVIEW TIMEFRAMES: NA

MCAT SCORES: 25.23

GPA: 3.5

IN-STATE TUITION: $46,627

OUT-OF-STATE TUITION: $46,627

TYPE OF SCHOOL: Private

DES MOINES UNIVERSITY

College of Osteopathic Medicine
3200 Grand Avenue
Des Moines, IA 50312-4198
Phone: 515-271-1451
Fax: 515-271-7163
doadmit@dmu.edu
www.dmu.edu

TOTAL ENROLLMENT: 819

% ACCEPTED: 18.20%

% MALE/FEMALE RATIO: 52/48

% UNDERREP. MINORITIES: 4%

APPLICATION DEADLINE: 2/1

APPLICATION NOTIFICATION: Rolling

EARLY APPLICATION DEADLINE: NA

EARLY APPLICATION NOTIFICATION: NA

TRANSFERS ACCEPTED: Yes

ADMISSIONS DEFFERABLE: Yes

APPLICATION FEE: $50

INTERVIEW TIMEFRAMES: NA

MCAT SCORES: 25.2

GPA: 3.56

IN-STATE TUITION: $45,950

OUT-OF-STATE TUITION: $45,950

TYPE OF SCHOOL: Private

Kansas City University of Medicine and Biosciences

College of Osteopathic Medicine
Office of Admissions
1750 Independence Avenue
Kansas City, MO 64106-1453
Phone: 800-234-4847
Fax: 816-460-0566
admissions@kcumb.edu
www.kcumb.edu

Total Enrollment: 887

% Accepted: 20.30%

% Male/female Ratio: 50/50

% Underrep. Minorities: 18%

Application Deadline: 2/6

Application Notification: Rolling

Early Application Deadline: Fall

Early Application Notification: 11/6

Transfers Accepted: No

Admissions Defferable: Yes

Application Fee: $50

Interview Timeframes: NA

MCAT Scores: 25.13

GPA: 3.54

In-state Tuition: $52,589

Out-of-state Tuition: $52,589

Type of School: Private

Lake Erie College of Osteopathic Medicine

Office of Admissions
1858 West Grandview Boulevard
Erie, PA 16509
Phone: 814-866-6641
Fax: 814-866-8123
admissions@lecom.edu
www.lcom.edu

Total Enrollment: 1206

% Accepted: NA

% Male/female Ratio: 54/46

% Underrep. Minorities: 8%

Application Deadline: 3/1

Application Notification: Rolling

Early Application Deadline: NA

Early Application Notification: NA

Transfers Accepted: No

Admissions Defferable: No

Application Fee: $50

Interview Timeframes: NA

MCAT Scores: NA

GPA: NA

In-state Tuition: $37,595

Out-of-state Tuition: $37,595

Type of School: Private

MICHIGAN STATE UNIVERSITY

College of Osteopathic Medicine
C110 East Fee Hall, MSUCOM
East Lansing, MI 48824-1316
Phone: 517-353-7740
Fax: 517-355-3296
comadm@com.msu.edu
www.com.msu.edu

TOTAL ENROLLMENT: 556

% ACCEPTED: 12%

% MALE/FEMALE RATIO: 54/46

% UNDERREP. MINORITIES: 6%

APPLICATION DEADLINE: 12/1

APPLICATION NOTIFICATION: Rolling

EARLY APPLICATION DEADLINE: 8/15

EARLY APPLICATION NOTIFICATION: 10/15

TRANSFERS ACCEPTED: Yes

ADMISSIONS DEFFERABLE: Yes

APPLICATION FEE: $75

INTERVIEW TIMEFRAMES: NA

MCAT SCORES: 24.9

GPA: 3.5

IN-STATE TUITION: $35,297

OUT-OF-STATE TUITION: $61,097

TYPE OF SCHOOL: Public

MIDWESTERN UNIVERSITY

Arizona College of Osteopathic Medicine
Office of Admissions
19555 North 59th Avenue
Glendale, AZ 85308
Phone: 623-572-3275
Fax: 623-572-3229
admissaz@arizona.midwestern.edu
www.midwestern.edu

TOTAL ENROLLMENT: 558

% ACCEPTED: 14.40%

% MALE/FEMALE RATIO: 63/37

% UNDERREP. MINORITIES: 54%

APPLICATION DEADLINE: 1/2

APPLICATION NOTIFICATION: 3/1

EARLY APPLICATION DEADLINE: NA

EARLY APPLICATION NOTIFICATION: NA

TRANSFERS ACCEPTED: Yes

ADMISSIONS DEFFERABLE: Yes

APPLICATION FEE: $50

INTERVIEW TIMEFRAMES: NA

MCAT SCORES: 26.7

GPA: 3.37

IN-STATE TUITION: $40,760

OUT-OF-STATE TUITION: $40,760

TYPE OF SCHOOL: Private

MIDWESTERN UNIVERSITY

Chicago College of Osteopathic Medicine
Office of Admissions
555 31st Street
Downers Grove, IL 60515
Phone: 800-458-6253
Fax: 630-971-6086
admissil@midwestern.edu
www.midwestern.edu

TOTAL ENROLLMENT: 690

% ACCEPTED: 11.90%

% MALE/FEMALE RATIO: 47/53

% UNDERREP. MINORITIES: 28%

APPLICATION DEADLINE: 1/1

APPLICATION NOTIFICATION: Rolling

EARLY APPLICATION DEADLINE: NA

EARLY APPLICATION NOTIFICATION: NA

TRANSFERS ACCEPTED: Yes

ADMISSIONS DEFFERABLE: Yes

APPLICATION FEE: $50

INTERVIEW TIMEFRAMES: NA

MCAT SCORES: 25.8

GPA: 3.5

IN-STATE TUITION: $45,358

OUT-OF-STATE TUITION: $45,358

TYPE OF SCHOOL: Private

NEW YORK INSTITUTE OF TECHNOLOGY

New York College of Osteopathic Medicine
Office of Admissions, NYCOM/NYIT
P.O. Box 8000
Old Westbury, NY 11568
Phone: 516-686-3747
Fax: 516-686-3831
admissions@nyit.edu
www.nyit.edu

TOTAL ENROLLMENT: NA

% ACCEPTED: NA

% MALE/FEMALE RATIO: 60/40

% UNDERREP. MINORITIES: 16%

APPLICATION DEADLINE: 2/1

APPLICATION NOTIFICATION: NA

EARLY APPLICATION DEADLINE: NA

EARLY APPLICATION NOTIFICATION: NA

TRANSFERS ACCEPTED: No

ADMISSIONS DEFFERABLE: No

APPLICATION FEE: NA

INTERVIEW TIMEFRAMES: November-May

MCAT SCORES: NA

GPA: NA

IN-STATE TUITION: $35,044

OUT-OF-STATE TUITION: $35,044

TYPE OF SCHOOL: Private

NOVA SOUTHEASTERN UNIVERSITY

College of Osteopathic Medicine
3200 South University Drive
Fort Lauderdale, FL 33328
Phone: 954-262-1101
Fax: 954-262-2282
com@nova.edu
www.medicine.nova.edu

TOTAL ENROLLMENT: 822

% ACCEPTED: 15.40%

% MALE/FEMALE RATIO: 50/50

% UNDERREP. MINORITIES: 32%

APPLICATION DEADLINE: 1/15

APPLICATION NOTIFICATION: Rolling

EARLY APPLICATION DEADLINE: NA

EARLY APPLICATION NOTIFICATION: NA

TRANSFERS ACCEPTED: Yes

ADMISSIONS DEFFERABLE: Yes

APPLICATION FEE: $50

INTERVIEW TIMEFRAMES: NA

MCAT SCORES: 25.01

GPA: 3.4

IN-STATE TUITION: $40,750

OUT-OF-STATE TUITION: $40,750

TYPE OF SCHOOL: Private

OHIO UNIVERSITY

College of Osteopathic Medicine
102 Grosvenor Hall
Athens, OH 45701
Phone: 800-345-1560
Fax: 740-593-2256
admissions@exchange.oucom.ohiou.edu
www.oucom.ohiou.edu

TOTAL ENROLLMENT: 433

% ACCEPTED: 6.70%

% MALE/FEMALE RATIO: 44/56

% UNDERREP. MINORITIES: 30%

APPLICATION DEADLINE: 2/6

APPLICATION NOTIFICATION: Rolling

EARLY APPLICATION DEADLINE: NA

EARLY APPLICATION NOTIFICATION: NA

TRANSFERS ACCEPTED: Yes

ADMISSIONS DEFFERABLE: Yes

APPLICATION FEE: $155

INTERVIEW TIMEFRAMES: NA

MCAT SCORES: 23.96

GPA: 3.54

IN-STATE TUITION: $43,919

OUT-OF-STATE TUITION: $53,351

TYPE OF SCHOOL: Public

OKLAHOMA STATE UNIVERSITY

College of Osteopathic Medicine
1111 West 17th Street
Office of Student Affairs
Tulsa, OK 74107
Phone: 918-561-8421
Fax: 918-561-8243
ldhaines@chs.okstate.edu
www.healthsciences.oksate.edu

TOTAL ENROLLMENT: 352

% ACCEPTED: 27.50%

% MALE/FEMALE RATIO: 53/47

% UNDERREP. MINORITIES: 18%

APPLICATION DEADLINE: 2/1

APPLICATION NOTIFICATION: Rolling

EARLY APPLICATION DEADLINE: NA

EARLY APPLICATION NOTIFICATION: NA

TRANSFERS ACCEPTED: Yes

ADMISSIONS DEFFERABLE: No

APPLICATION FEE: $25

INTERVIEW TIMEFRAMES: November-April

MCAT SCORES: 26

GPA: 3.59

IN-STATE TUITION: $27,638

OUT-OF-STATE TUITION: $42,858

TYPE OF SCHOOL: Public

PHILADELPHIA COLLEGE OF OSTEOPATHIC MEDICINE

Office of Admissions
4170 City Avenue
Philadelphia, PA 19131
Phone: 800-999-6998
Fax: 215-871-6719
admissions@pcom.edu
www.pcom.edu

TOTAL ENROLLMENT: 1041

% ACCEPTED: 15%

% MALE/FEMALE RATIO: 47/53

% UNDERREP. MINORITIES: 23%

APPLICATION DEADLINE: 2/1

APPLICATION NOTIFICATION: Rolling

EARLY APPLICATION DEADLINE: NA

EARLY APPLICATION NOTIFICATION: NA

TRANSFERS ACCEPTED: No

ADMISSIONS DEFFERABLE: No

APPLICATION FEE: $50

INTERVIEW TIMEFRAMES: NA

MCAT SCORES: 24.39

GPA: 3.34

IN-STATE TUITION: $44,165

OUT-OF-STATE TUITION: $44,165

TYPE OF SCHOOL: Private

PIKEVILLE COLLEGE

School of Osteopathic Medicine
147 Sycamore Street
Pikeville, KY 41501
Phone: 606-218-5406
Fax: 606-218-5405
ahamilto@pc.edu

www.pcsom.edu

TOTAL ENROLLMENT: 278

% ACCEPTED: 9.60%

% MALE/FEMALE RATIO: 57/43

% UNDERREP. MINORITIES: 5%

APPLICATION DEADLINE: 2/5

APPLICATION NOTIFICATION: Rolling

EARLY APPLICATION DEADLINE: NA

EARLY APPLICATION NOTIFICATION: NA

TRANSFERS ACCEPTED: Yes

ADMISSIONS DEFFERABLE: Yes

APPLICATION FEE: $75

INTERVIEW TIMEFRAMES: NA

MCAT SCORES: 21.7

GPA: 3.31

IN-STATE TUITION: $35,000

OUT-OF-STATE TUITION: $35,000

TYPE OF SCHOOL: Private

TOURO UNIVERSITY—CALIFORNIA

College of Osteopathic Medicine
Office of Admissions
1310 Johnson Lane
Vallejo, CA 94592
Phone: 707-638-5270
Fax: 707-638-5250
sdavis@touro.edu

www.tu.edu

TOTAL ENROLLMENT: 525

% ACCEPTED: 4.10%

% MALE/FEMALE RATIO: 53/47

% UNDERREP. MINORITIES: 5%

APPLICATION DEADLINE: 4/1

APPLICATION NOTIFICATION: Rolling

EARLY APPLICATION DEADLINE: 8/15

EARLY APPLICATION NOTIFICATION: 9/15

TRANSFERS ACCEPTED: Yes

ADMISSIONS DEFFERABLE: Yes

APPLICATION FEE: $100

INTERVIEW TIMEFRAMES: NA

MCAT SCORES: 26.25

GPA: 3.3

IN-STATE TUITION: $36,694

OUT-OF-STATE TUITION: $36,694

TYPE OF SCHOOL: Private

University of Medicine and Dentistry of New Jersey

School of Osteopathic Medicine
1 Medical Center Drive, Suite 210
Stratford, NJ 08084
Phone: 856-566-7050
Fax: 856-566-6895
somadm@umdnj.edu

som.umdnj.edu

Total Enrollment: 382

% Accepted: 12.10%

% Male/female Ratio: 43/57

% Underrep. Minorities: 53%

Application Deadline: 2/1

Application Notification: Rolling

Early Application Deadline: NA

Early Application Notification: NA

Transfers Accepted: Yes

Admissions Defferable: Yes

Application Fee: $75

Interview Timeframes: NA

MCAT Scores: 26.7

GPA: 3.5

In-state Tuition: $42,513

Out-of-state Tuition: $54,595

Type of School: Public

University of New England

College of Osteopathic Medicine
UNECOM Recruitment
Student & Alumni Services
11 Hills Beach Road
Phone: 207-602-2329
Fax: 207-602-5967
unecomadmissions@une.edu

www.une.edu/com

Total Enrollment: 500

% Accepted: 9%

% Male/female Ratio: 48/52

% Underrep. Minorities: 10%

Application Deadline: 2/1

Application Notification: Rolling

Early Application Deadline: NA

Early Application Notification: NA

Transfers Accepted: Yes

Admissions Defferable: No

Application Fee: $55

Interview Timeframes: September-April

MCAT Scores: 24.97

GPA: 3.37

In-state Tuition: $50,180

Out-of-state Tuition: $50,180

Type of School: Private

UNIVERSITY OF NORTH TEXAS HEALTH SCIENCE CENTER

Texas College of Osteopathic Medicine
Office of Admissions & Outreach, EAD-248
3500 Camp Bowie Boulevard
Forth Worth, TX 76107-2699
Phone: 817-735-2204
Fax: 817-735-2225
tcomadmissions@hsc.unt.edu

www.hsc.unt.edu/education/tcom/
admissions.cfm

TOTAL ENROLLMENT: 520

% ACCEPTED: 10.40%

% MALE/FEMALE RATIO: 47/53

% UNDERREP. MINORITIES: 10%

APPLICATION DEADLINE: 10/15

APPLICATION NOTIFICATION: 7/20

EARLY APPLICATION DEADLINE: 5/1

EARLY APPLICATION NOTIFICATION: 10/15

TRANSFERS ACCEPTED: Yes

ADMISSIONS DEFFERABLE: Yes

APPLICATION FEE: NA

INTERVIEW TIMEFRAMES: August-December

MCAT SCORES: 27.5

GPA: 3.5

IN-STATE TUITION: $24,107

OUT-OF-STATE TUITION: $39,857

TYPE OF SCHOOL: Public

VIRGINIA COLLEGE OF OSTEOPATHIC MEDICINE (VCOM)

Edward Via Virginia College of
Osteopathic Medicine
Office of Admissions, VCOM
2265 Kraft Drive
Blacksburg, VA 24060
Phone: 540-231-6138
Fax: 540-231-5252
admissions@vcom.vt.edu

www.vcom.vt.edu

TOTAL ENROLLMENT: 610

% ACCEPTED: 11.70%

% MALE/FEMALE RATIO: 51/49

% UNDERREP. MINORITIES: 13%

APPLICATION DEADLINE: 2/7

APPLICATION NOTIFICATION: 12/6

EARLY APPLICATION DEADLINE: 9/6

EARLY APPLICATION NOTIFICATION: 10/6

TRANSFERS ACCEPTED: Yes

ADMISSIONS DEFFERABLE: Yes

APPLICATION FEE: $75

INTERVIEW TIMEFRAMES: NA

MCAT SCORES: 24

GPA: 3.5

IN-STATE TUITION: $55,450

OUT-OF-STATE TUITION: $55,450

TYPE OF SCHOOL: Private

West Virginia School of Osteopathic Medicine

Director of Admissions
400 North Lee Street
Lewisburg, WV 24901
Phone: 800-356-7836
Fax: 304-645-4859
admissions@wvsom.edu

www.wvsom.edu

Total Enrollment: 397

% Accepted: 19%

% Male/female Ratio: 53/47

% Underrep. Minorities: 11%

Application Deadline: 2/1

Application Notification: Rolling

Early Application Deadline: 11/1

Early Application Notification: 12/6

Transfers Accepted: Yes

Admissions Defferable: Yes

Application Fee: $155

Interview Timeframes: August-April

MCAT Scores: 21.9

GPA: 3.48

In-state Tuition: $35,430

Out-of-state Tuition: $61,458

Type of School: Public

Western University of Health Sciences

College of Osteopathic Medicine of the Pacific
Office of Admissions
Pomona, CA 91766-1854
Phone: 909-469-5335
Fax: 909-469-5570
admissions@westernu.edu

www.westernu.edu

Total Enrollment: 724

% Accepted: 23.20%

% Male/female Ratio: 50/50

% Underrep. Minorities: 46%

Application Deadline: 3/1

Application Notification: Rolling

Early Application Deadline: NA

Early Application Notification: NA

Transfers Accepted: Yes

Admissions Defferable: Yes

Application Fee: $65

Interview Timeframes: NA

MCAT Scores: 26.53

GPA: 3.47

In-state Tuition: $48,440

Out-of-state Tuition: $48,440

Type of School: Private

Notes

Notes

Notes

Notes

About the Authors

Dr. Mohan had the rare happenstance of getting into every medical school she applied to. She attributes this mostly to her adventurous personal statements, including how her greatest achievement was making caramel fudge brownies (not to mention she got accepted to Pomona College with an essay on the cartoon Pinky & the Brain). She served on the admissions committees at Cornell Medical College and at UC Berkeley's School of Public Health, where she received her Master's in International Health Policy & Development. This experience, combined with 12 years of teaching (6 years of MCAT and personal statement consulting) provided the insights presented in this book. Currently, Dr. Mohan is the VP of Wellness Programming at an IPTV broadcast network, and is pursuing her credentials in ayurvedic medicine. She also has a blog devoted to an "east meets west" approach to health (www.svasthahealth.com). To contact Dr. Mohan, please visit her website at www.raakhimohan.com.

Dr. Busnaina had the bizarre experience of only securing admission offers to top 5 medical schools despite having applied "across the board." Amidst the perplexion, he entered medical school only to find he was too young to take part in many of the over-21 orientation activities. While at the University of Pennsylvania, he was one of the only medical students to develop contacts and arrange his own international clinical and research rotations, which was considered fairly unusual at the time. His successful experience in the medical school admissions process, as well as that for MBA, PhD, and Master's programs, was the the source of his inspiration and insight into writing this book. Currently, Dr. Busnaina is a resident at the University of California, Los Angeles, and works as a physician consultant at the Hollywood, Health & Society project at the University of Southern California, working with writers of top television programs in delivering accurate health messages and evaluating the impact of those messages on their audiences.